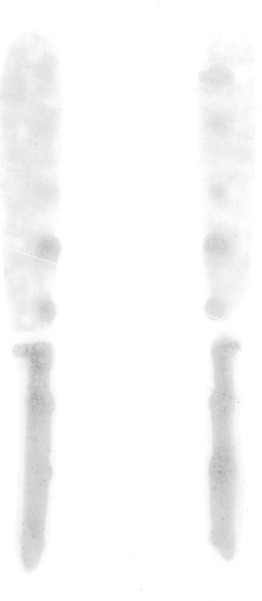

The Artificial Face

The Artificial Face

A History of Cosmetics

Fenja Gunn

with drawings by the author

HIPPOCRENE
BOOKS, INC.

Hippocrene Books, Inc.
171 Madison Avenue
New York, N.Y. 10016

ISBN 0-88254-272-9

Library of Congress Catalog Card Number 74-80438

Printed in Great Britain

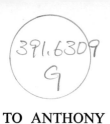

TO ANTHONY

CONTENTS

LIST OF ILLUSTRATIONS

9

LIST OF ILLUSTRATIONS

facing page

DRAWINGS

DRAWINGS

28; Dr Andrew Strathern, 2; Victoria & Albert Museum, 17, 35; *Vogue* Magazine, Condé Nast Publications Ltd, 42; Yardley & Co Ltd, 40.

DRAWINGS listed above are reproduced by courtesy of the following: Martin Battersby Esq, 26; Brighton Museum and Art Gallery, 14, 17; British Museum, 1, 2, 3, 4, 5, 6, 7, 8; David Crook Esq, 27; Harvey Daniels Esq, 29; Hampshire County Museum Service, Winchester, 30; Edmund Launert Esq, 23; Trustees of the London Museum, 19; Mrs Betty O'Looney, 28; The Pitt-Rivers Museum, 20; Private collection, 24; Victoria & Albert Museum, 9, 10, 11, 12, 13, 15, 18, 21; The Welcome Trustees, 16; Yardley & Co Ltd, 22, 25.

All the drawings are by the author.

Foreword

The aim of this book is to illustrate, through a history of cosmetic fashions, the changing ideals of beauty at different historical periods. A detailed study of the daily toilet of both men and women through the ages allows one to observe changes in moral attitudes and social conditions, as well as the influences of positive events, such as wars or revolutions, which alter the whole climate of a period.

The particular appeal of a historical study of this nature is found in intimate detail and I felt, therefore, that it was essential to narrow down my field of research to one country. Thus, the main part of the book is devoted to the history of cosmetics in England. Although there have been several encyclopaedic or technical works on the subject and other books have described the make-up fashions of a number of countries, very few have dealt specifically with the *toilette* of English men and women.

The first three chapters of *The Artificial Face* are intended as an introduction to the main part of the book. Chapter 1 deals with the origins of cosmetics in prehistoric body and face painting, illustrated by examples from primitive societies. Chapters 2 and 3 describe the beauty preparations and customs of the ancient Middle Eastern and Mediterranean civilisations. These early cultures had a positive and continuing influence on the cosmetics and make-up fashions of European countries, including England.

The book covers every aspect of the appearance relating to the 'artificial face', including hair styles, and also observes the development of hygiene and perfumery.

Many books on beauty are written expressly or subconsciously in sympathy with the fashion ideal of the period they describe. In *The Artificial Face* I have attempted to reveal fashionable beauty through the eyes of painter and caricaturist alike, and through the writings of both fashion followers and puritan reformists. My intention has been that the fashionable face should be viewed three-dimensionally and from every possible, even if unflattering, angle. Material for the book has been gathered from a number of contemporary sources, including chronicles, diaries, recipe books, drama, prose and poetry. The pen-and-ink drawings illustrate the type of cosmetic containers or toilet implements common to particular periods of history. I have thus sought to reproduce the individual character of each century, an intrinsic requirement of any study as specialised as a history of cosmetics.

F.G.

PART ONE

Introduction

CHAPTER ONE

The Origins of Cosmetics

Primitive art is a practical instrument for the important business of daily living. (R. Arnheim, *Art and Visual Perception: A Psychology of the Creative Eye*, 1960)

Throughout recorded history cosmetics have been used to create the beauty ideal of each passing age and for centuries a daily routine of beauty care has been an accepted 'ritual' within a social context. Women and even men, it seems, have always had a fascination for changing their appearance with the aid of paints, powders, dyes, depilatory devices and other artificial methods, and the general acceptance of this practice as a manifestation of civilised living has disguised its ancient pagan origins.

The use of cosmetics, far from being a product of civilisation, originates from an inherent and primitive human need for self-decoration. As far back as 100,000 BC, Neanderthal man is believed to have painted his body and practised tattooing, the earliest form of 'cosmetic' mutilation; and, at a later period, the men of the New Stone Age are thought to have decorated their bodies in a similar fashion. However, the original motivation behind prehistoric man's use of paint was quite different from that which inspired civilised cultures to adopt cosmetic artifice as a means of enhancing or creating beauty.

Prehistoric man must have been conscious that he was a

weak animal in a totally hostile environment. As a hunter he had to develop his own tools of aggression because Nature had not provided him with sharp teeth or claws or the overwhelming physical strength of the wild beasts which roamed the ancient world. He was overawed and dominated by the elements and a prey to countless fears engendered by the apparently mysterious works of Nature. This prompted him to seek some form of environmental camouflage and it is reasonable to assume that he chose to disguise his human identity with paint. There are numerous examples of this type of 'camouflage' existing in primitive societies, and prehistoric men undoubtedly used body painting for the same reasons as the Australian aboriginal, the African tribesman or the North American Indian. First it was used as a means of blending with the natural environment while hunting or tracking prey; secondly as a means of stimulating fear in an aggressive confrontation, and thirdly for spiritual and social reasons. In all these cases primitive man exhibits his fear of the natural environment and, paradoxically, his desire to dominate it by aggression or, failing this, to come to terms with it by placation.

He painted the markings of the most powerful animals on his own skin because he believed that by representing their physical characteristics on his body he acquired some of their power. This magical strength could then be used spiritually to dominate creatures of the animal world and to impress his own kind. But his fear of wild beasts and his surroundings remained as a constantly disturbing and inexplicable phenomenon, and inspired primitive man with the belief that mysterious forces were at work around him which he could neither understand nor control. As a result he gave these forces tangible substance by personifying them as gods. These deities of the primitive world took the shape of wild beasts, birds and reptiles imbued by man with mysterious powers over the environment. The trees, wind, sun and stars also had a spiritual significance for primitive humans, and worship of these powers took the form of communal ritual in which the gods were placated with gifts and promises of loyalty in return for their protection of the tribe.

Body and face painting played an essential part in these ceremonies as it was used as a form of stage make-up by dancers and singers enacting specific magical roles within the ritual (*Plate 1*). Different patterns and colours were used to define these roles and each primitive tribe developed its own design forms which varied according to the ceremonial. These decorative patterns were frequently an abstract representation of the tribal totem, the animal or bird spirit which was adopted by the community to protect its members from the aggression of another tribe or the spectral forces of evil. The totem spirit acted as an intermediary between man and nature and its symbolic form once painted on the body acted as a 'spiritual armour'. As primitive communities developed in size and social complexity, different totems were adopted by clan groups or individuals as a means of establishing their identity or status within the society. Thus decorative body or tattoo patterns increased in variety.

Colour also gave a specific character to body and face paintings, and it is obvious that, at an early stage in the world's development, men were aware of the effect colour can have on the human emotions. Some anthropologists believe that prehistoric man first responded to the colours of the solar spectrum, before blues and greens, because the sun represented a powerful force which brought daylight and safety from the real and imaginary dangers of night time. Among primitive peoples red and yellow paints still have a special emotional significance. The Australian aborigines regard yellow as the colour of peace and all primitive communities use red body paint for important ceremonials. The people of Mount Hagen in New Guinea colour their skins with red ochre for festive rituals which celebrate victory in battle or success in commercial exchange, and most

21

native tribes use red body dyes for initiation rites and burial ceremonies and also as a sign of aggression in warfare. In many cases red paint symbolically represents blood and it is believed that primitive man, even in prehistory, used it on the bones of corpses to effect 'reanimation' after death. Black and white dyes are also much used in body decoration; black paint, which symbolises night time and darkness, is frequently employed in rituals of a sinister or aggressive character, whereas white paint represents the amorphous nature of the spiritual world.

The domination of primitive peoples by their environment is evident from the fact that daily life, ritual and nature are inextricably intermingled and, as in the animal kingdom, different moods are conveyed by physical display. Painted patterns and graphic application of colour on the face and body are used in primitive societies to create the right atmosphere for every occasion. Thus, some tribal peoples have developed a whole language of 'cosmetic' art with which to express their feelings. Coloured designs, tattoos, the use of oils and fragrances or even hairstyling are all employed to enhance a mood, convey a meaning or define a social or sexual condition.

The Mount Hagen people of New Guinea use dyes to differentiate between male and female elements in ritual ceremonies (*Plate 2*). Black paint represents male aggression and hidden strength, whereas red defines the female element, signifying magic, friendliness, material wealth and fertility. Girls during courtship use hair oil and paint a band of charcoal or red dye across their foreheads, and decorate their faces with spots and triangles of colour. Men decorate their features with red, yellow, blue and white patterns, which are echoed again in the magnificent painted wigs they wear as a symbol of male potency. These edifices of hair and the bright colours of courtship are immediately rejected during a period of mourning, when the well-oiled bodies of both sexes are smeared with ashes and mud to give the opposite effect to a shining polished skin. Australian aborigines have an elaborate system of colouring during a mourning period. A man paints his face and torso if his wife or brother-in-law dies and a woman does the same after the death of her husband. Black paint is used for a death in one's own generation, whereas red is the colour used for parents of the children's generation.

Various stages of physical development are also marked by the use of paint or 'cosmetic' devices. The people of Nuba in the Sudan use a particular hair style and body scarification to indicate that a child has reached the age of eight or nine, and in many tribes puberty is marked by initiation rites which include ritual painting and tattooing of the body. The pain inflicted on the initiate by the execution of these tattoos is an essential part of the ceremony, but in many societies tattoos are considered an aid to beauty in their own right.

The elaborate forms of 'cosmetic mutilation' found in native communities, such as tattooing, plucking out facial and body hair, filing teeth and deliberate deformation of physical features, also find their parallels in civilised cultures. The extraordinary idea that one 'must suffer to be beautiful' may well originate from the primitive initiation ceremony in which the initiate had to suffer 'cosmetic mutilation' to justify his manhood. At any rate, the eyebrow tweezer has remained throughout history as the most universally popular cosmetic implement, and the painful plucking out of facial hair has been practised in civilised societies for centuries.

Undoubtedly personal vanity and a desire to appear attractive to the opposite sex are important reasons for cosmetic decoration. Painting and tattooing for ritual may have been the original purpose of cosmetic art, but the simple human need to attract sexually those of one's own kind cannot be excluded as a motivation. In primitive communities face paint and the use of oils and fragrance are all employed to create physical desirability as they have been in cultured societies, and in many cases the 'beauty' effects which they are designed to achieve are also similar. Paints are used to emphasise the eyes and highlight facial characteristics; black dyes are employed to enhance the beauty of a dark skin in the same way that white face powder is used to create a pale complexion. Red ochre powder is employed as a face colourant and for many centuries it was used as a rouge by civilised cultures. Other natural materials, such as chalk and powdered limestone, are employed in the manufacture of face paints by primitive and cultured societies alike. Animal and vegetable oils, used in their natural state by native tribes, form the basis for many sophisticated beauty preparations, and toilet implements, such as 'make-up brushes' made from twigs and leaf swabs, are primitive editions of those used today. Fragrant leaves, flowers and aromatic substances are substitutes, in native societies, for perfumes or scented pomades.

Hairstyling is of equal importance to civilised and primitive peoples. Judging from the numerous pins and ornaments which have been found dating from the Neolithic period, interest in the hair dates from prehistory. In some native societies, abundant tresses symbolise male potency and in other cases the styling, shaving or cutting of hair has a ritual significance.

However, for both sexes, a carefully nurtured and styled 'coiffure' is a desirable feature of beauty. Beeswax, resins and oils are used as dressings or conditioners; 'permanent waving' techniques are employed to straighten the hair using sticks and paste, and urine is used amongst primitive Indians as an effective bleach. Elaborate wigs made from natural fibres or hair are worn by many native peoples to provide supplementary tresses.

In primitive societies the dependence on ritual influenced the whole performance of personal grooming and application of cosmetic paints. These followed set conventions whether used for ceremonial or social purposes, and the toilet became in its own right a form of ritual which occupied a particular period of each day, as time was needed to achieve 'cosmetic' perfection and an artificial ideal of beauty.

Thus the daily creation of physical desirability by artifice has become an essential part of everyday life in cultured societies, and cosmetics which originated from paints used by primitive man in prehistory to disguise his human appearance have become an accepted form of social camouflage which stereotypes facial characteristics into an image of beauty that varies with the passage of time.

CHAPTER TWO

Cosmetics in Antiquity: The Middle East

Her lips are enchantment,
　her neck the right length
　　and her breasts a marvel;
Her hair lapislazuli in its glitter,
　her arms more splendid than gold.
　Her fingers make me see petals,
　　The lotus' are like that
(*Love Poems of Ancient Egypt*, translated from Ancient Egyptian
Papyri by Ezra Pound and Noel Stock)

The magical origins of body and face painting continued to influence the early Middle Eastern and Mediterranean civilisations in their use of face paints, aromatics and ritual cleansing as an intrinsic part of religious rites; and the ancient mystical significance of self decoration affected the attitudes of these civilisations to artificial beauty. It is an interesting fact that all the early cultured peoples accentuated the eye, giving it prominence over any other feature of the face. The importance of the eye in antiquity has its origin in an ancient heritage of pagan religion, superstition and magic. It has always been referred to as the mirror of a man's soul and in the ancient world was a symbol of both good and evil. It was painted on ships to guide them through troubled seas to safety. In ancient Egypt it was the symbol of the sun god Re and in most early writings it

26

appears as a significant hieroglyphic device. It was thus logical that the human eye should be given a special importance by accentuation with cosmetic paints, thereby imbuing it with the mystical quality of a sacred emblem.

The dominance of the eye as a symbol of beauty is clearly seen in the frescoes and painted human images of ancient Egypt. The perfect state of preservation of these images provides a vivid picture of these people of antiquity. The sensuous vitality of Tutankhamun and the handsome arrogance of Ankhenaten represent masculine ideals in appearance, and the cool elegance of Nefertiti has a timeless quality of feminine beauty. The Egyptians were a handsome people with symmetrically formed features and richly bronzed faces framed by sculptured wigs of ebony hair. Their appearance was rendered even more exotic by the extravagant nature of their eye make-up. The dark almond-shaped eyes of both sexes were ringed with a dark green cosmetic or outlined with black paint drawn into winged lines at the end corner of the eye (*Plate 3*).

The origin of Egyptian eye-paint, or *msdmt* as it was called, is not clearly known. There is evidence of the importation of eye make-up from China during the twelfth and eighteenth dynasties, and other evidence is provided by a fresco which shows an Egyptian nobleman receiving a present of eye-paint from the Aamu people of western Asia. Raw materials for manufacturing this make-up were available in Egypt; the Far East and western Asia may simply have been alternative sources for this cosmetic commodity rather than its places of origin.

Egyptian eye make-up predominantly consisted of malachite, a green ore of copper, and galena, a dark grey ore of lead. Malachite was the earlier form of eye-paint and was obtained in its raw state from Sinai and the eastern desert, whilst galena was found near Aswan and the Red Sea coast. Other materials for eye-paint, or kohl, included carbonate of lead, oxide of

27

copper, iron and manganese, brown ochre, chrysocolla—a greenish-blue copper ore—and sulphide of antimony. All these materials were obtained locally with the exception of antimony which was imported from Asia Minor, Persia and possibly Arabia.

Eye-paint was prepared by grinding the raw materials on a stone slab or palette after which the compound was placed in a container. Shells, hollow reeds and small alabaster vases were used to contain kohl until it was needed, when it was probably mixed with animal fat or a vegetable oil. It was also applied in powder form over a base of ointment; but in either case a wooden or ivory stick was used to paint the cosmetic substance

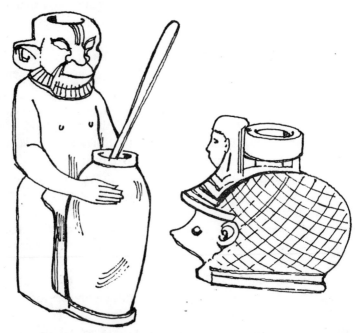

Fig 1 (*left*) glazed composition kohl-pot, with wooden kohl stick, held by the god Bes, *c* 600 BC; (*right*) glazed composition cosmetic pot in the shape of a hedgehog, *c* 600 BC

28

round the eyes. The underside of the lid was frequently painted with green malachite whilst the upper lid, lashes and brows were darkened with galena.

Apart from the decorative value of this exotic eye-paint, there is evidence that it was used for medicinal purposes. A copper substance used in the paint guarded against suppuration of the eyes due to the intense glare of the sun and acted as a preventive measure against eye diseases which were prevalent during the

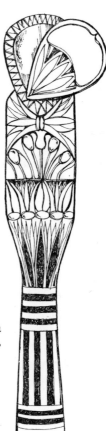

Fig 2 Wooden ointment spoon in the shape of a bouquet of lotus flowers with buds of tinted ivory, *c* 1300 BC

29

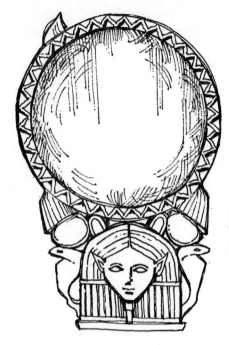

Fig 3 Ivory ointment spoon
with carved handle in the
shape of a Hathor head and
two uraei, *c* 1300BC

period of the Nile's inundation. For this reason children as
well as men and women were encouraged to use kohl.

Once her eyes were decoratively painted, the aristocratic
Egyptian woman would have turned her attention to the rest of
her toilet. Her cheeks and lips would have been dyed with a
mixture of red ochre combined with fat or oil and, in the case of
the rouge, a little gum resin was added as an ingredient. The
palms of her hands and her finger nails were reddened with a
dye made from henna, and the nipples of her breasts were gilded
with gold paint. Cleansing creams, used to preserve her skin in
good condition, were made from animal or vegetable oil mixed
with lime or chalk, and soothing ointments were compounded
of fat, wax and powdered limestone. These cosmetic concoctions were always scented with crushed flower petals, aromatic

30

spices and perfumes to render them pleasant to use. Aristocratic men also made use of the same wide range of cosmetic materials, especially aromatic oils and ointments.

Another aspect of the toilet which was of prime importance to the ancient Egyptians was the use of depilatory devices to rid their bodies and heads of hair. 'Egyptians are shaven at other times, but after a death they let their hair and beard grow.' (Herodotus.) Depilatory creams, razors and pumice stones were used for this purpose; both sexes shaved themselves bald and wore elaborate wigs. These were dyed ebony black or dark red with henna, and made from human hair dressed with beeswax, flax, wool or palm fibre. The poorer classes had to be content with felt. The wigs worn by the aristocracy were braided and plaited into shape and frequently embellished with exotic jewellery, but the most magnificent wigs adorned the Pharaohs who also wore plaited false beards on ceremonial occasions. During the reign of the heretic Pharaoh, Ankhenaten, wigs became particularly flamboyant. Men wore vast curled concoctions and women adorned themselves with top heavy edifices of hair festooned with long plaited artificial tresses (*Plate 4*).

The fashion for this total lack of natural hair undoubtedly stemmed from an understandable obsession with hygiene. The high temperatures reached in the Nile valley encouraged germs and diseases to breed. The shaving of all body hair was an excellent preventive measure against infection whilst maintaining a degree of comfort in the hot Middle Eastern weather. The Egyptians are reputed to have bathed several times a day and Herodotus states that 'they set cleanness above seemliness'. Each bath or douche was followed by liberal applications of perfumes and unguents, and guests were offered the courtesy of having their feet and hands bathed and scented with aromatic oils. Their heads were also anointed with sweet smelling perfumes.

Perfumery was yet another aspect of the Egyptian toilet which, like the use of eye-paint, had its roots in mysticism and magic. The preparation of aromatic scents was, in the early stages of Egyptian civilisation, entirely the specialist preserve of priests, who used aromatics as an essential part of religious ceremonies and in the process of embalming. Sacrificial oxen were disembowelled and filled 'with pure bread, honey, raisins, figs, frankincense, myrrh, and other kinds of incense . . .' (Herodotus), whilst the corpses of humans were rinsed out with palm wine and crushed spices after which their empty stomachs were filled with 'pure ground myrrh and cassia and any other spices, save only frankincense . . .' (Herodotus.) Wealthy aristocrats were injected with aromatic cedar oil through the body orifices.

The use of perfumes in priestly ritual imbued scent with a special magical significance and is probably the reason why Egyptian perfumed cosmetics were held in such esteem by the rest of the civilised world during the course of ancient history. Egyptian scented oils and unguents were prepared from a variety of natural ingredients, including myrrh, cinnamon, cassia, cardamon, spikenard, iris root, honey, wine, aromatic resins and scented woods. The process of perfume distillation had not been invented, so all scents were based on fat or oil to ensure a degree of fixation. Sesame, almond, olive and castor oil were used and 'balanos' oil, which was extracted from the shells of some unknown fruit, was also favoured in the manufacture of unguents. An important centre for aromatic cosmetics was Mendes, and raw materials for ointments and oils were imported from the Greek islands and other sources in the Middle East. One of the most famous Mendesian unguents was a mixture of 'balanos' oil, myrrh, cassia and gum resin, and this compound was greatly favoured by ancient Egyptian society.

Perfumes and unguents frequently contained medicinal properties and it is interesting to note that the Egyptian queen, Cleopatra, is reputed to have combined her considerable talents to produce a book on beauty preparations and an advanced

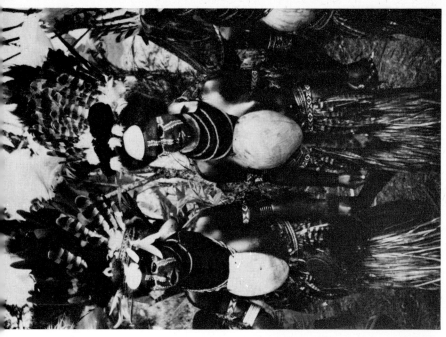

and face painting, from south-eastern Nuba in the Sudan. Black and yellow paints are used to achieve this bold effect. The eyes are clearly emphasised—in common with make-up fashions of cultured societies.

2 (*right*) Two young women from Mount Hagen in New Guinea dressed in full regalia with feathered head-dresses. The ceremonial face painting is of white and blue dye on a bright red foundation.

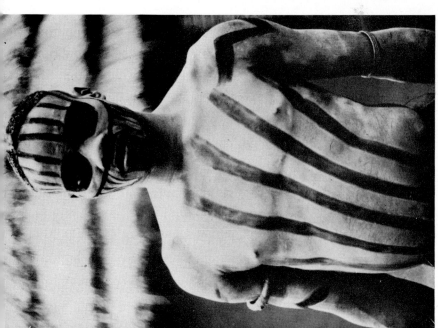

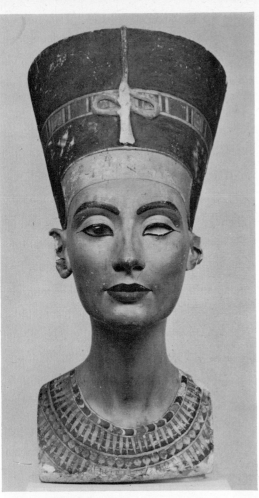

3 (*left*) Bust of Queen Nefertiti. Her exotic eye-paint is a good example of the kind of eye decoration used by both men and women of ancient Egypt. The lips are rouged.

4 (*below left*) Wall frieze from the tomb of Nebamun, Thebes, illustrates the elaborate hair styles (most probably wigs) of ancient Egyptian society. The eyes are painted in the distinctive fashion resemble the sacred eye of Re.

5 (*below right*) The head of Ashurnasirpal, King of Nimrud. The stylised treatment of the hair and beard nevertheless indicates t employment of artificial curling devices. The use of eye-paint is similar to that of ancient Egypt.

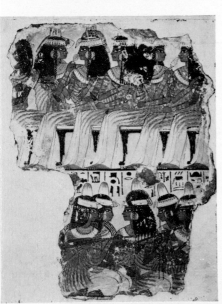

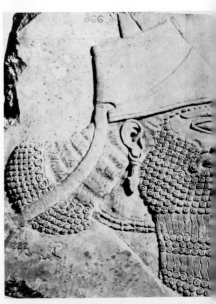

treatise on alchemy. However, her cure for baldness is of a somewhat dubious nature: 'For bald patches, powder red sulphuret of arsenic and take it up with oak gum, as much as it will bear. Put on a rag and apply, having soaped the place well first. I have mixed the above with foam of nitre and it worked well.' (Galen.) Although baldness was desirable during many stages of Egyptian civilisation, at the much later date of Cleopatra's reign, hair was once more in fashion.

The sophistication of Egyptian cosmetics was only eclipsed by the advanced design of the beauty equipment. Mirrors of polished metal have been discovered in tombs dating from the sixth dynasty, about 2800 BC, and kohl vases of glass which date from 1500 BC. Queen Hetepheres, the mother of the Pharaoh who was reputed to have built the great pyramid of Giza, was provided for her after-life with thirty alabaster cosmetic vessels and a beautiful toilet box of eight inscribed alabaster jars, plus a whole range of toilet implements in gold, copper and flint. Exquisite cosmetic containers were found in the tomb of Tutankhamun, including a make-up chest in cedar and ivory inlaid with black pigments, plated in silver and gold and decorated with magical symbols. An unusually beautiful mirror box was also discovered, designed in the shape of the *ankh* symbol of life and plated in gold with a silver edging. Alternative containers included an ebony chest for antimony powder and a selection of beautifully fashioned alabaster jars which were still haunted with the elusive fragrance of unguents dating from about 1350 BC. Other tomb excavations have yielded a wealth of cosmetic implements, such as manicure tools and razors, made of gold.

The Egyptians were known throughout the ancient world for their cosmetic skills. Trade with Egypt introduced paint and perfume to many Middle Eastern peoples, among them the Hebrews. There is no evidence of the use of aromatics in Israel until after Abram's journey to Egypt, described in the Book of

Genesis, although it is obvious that Semitic tribes imported aromatics and spices into the Nile valley. 'And they sat down to eat bread: and they lifted up their eyes and looked, and, behold, a company of Ishmaelites came from Gilead with their camels bearing spicery, and balm and myrrh, going to carry it down to Egypt.' (Genesis 37:25.)

After the introduction of aromatics into Israel through Egypt, the Hebrew people evidently acquired a taste for perfume as there are repeated references to scent in the Bible. In the Book of Exodus (25:6), the description of religious ceremonial relating to the Holy Tabernacle alludes to the use of spiced oils and incense as an essential part of the holy ritual: 'Oil for the light, spices for anointing oil, and for sweet incense'; and in the beautiful Song of Solomon there are many references to the aesthetic qualities of perfume used in a purely secular context.

> While the King sitteth at his table my Spikenard sendeth forth the smell thereof. A bundle of myrrh is my well-beloved unto me; he shall lie all night betwixt my breasts. My beloved is unto me as a cluster of camphire in the vineyards of En-ge-di.
>
> (1:12, 13, 14)

Cosmetics were also employed by many Hebrew women to enhance their looks, although this practice was not generally approved by Jewish prophets and a puritan element in Hebrew society. 'And when thou art spoiled, what wilt thou do? though thou clothest thyself with crimson, though thou deckedst thee with ornaments of gold, though thou rentest thy face with painting, in vain shalt thou make thyself fair; thy lovers will despise thee, they will seek thy life.' (Jeremiah 4:30.)

The most famous 'painted' woman in the Bible is undoubtedly Jezebel, who adorned her face with cosmetic paints and dramatised her eyes with the use of kohl in order to appear seductive: 'And when Jehu was come to Jezebel, Jezebel heard of it; and she painted her face, and tired her head, and looked out at a window.' (Kings 9:30.)

34

Apart from the influence of Egyptian cosmetic devices on Hebrew women, the neighbouring Mesopotamian cultures also employed the use of paints and perfumes, and as the Jewish people were in contact with these civilisations it is likely that they were influenced by the Babylonian and Assyrian mode of dress and self-decoration.

The Mesopotamian peoples shared a basic similarity in appearance. Their exotic clothing emphasised the sultry beauty of their dark skins and the proud hawk-like features of men and women were enhanced by a luxuriant growth of blue-black hair. Unlike the Egyptians, the Mesopotamians of both sexes grew their hair to nearly waist length, after which it was elaborately dressed and artificially curled into extravagant styles. Women coiled their locks into a chignon, and men dressed their hair in a similar fashion with two braided tresses crossing underneath the chignon and fastening over the forehead. Beards were tightly curled into numerous shell-like whorls and were frequently interwoven with gold thread (*Plate 5*). Both sexes dressed their locks with aromatic oils, scented them with perfume and, if a variation in colour was desired, used dyes made from cedar oil, alum and anthemis.

Facial cosmetics were also used by the Mesopotamians. One of the earliest examples of lip salve was discovered during the excavation of Ur, capital city of the Chaldeans. This cosmetic was prepared from a base of white lead and dates back to approximately 3500 BC. Self-decoration also extended to the eyes which were accentuated with paints and the brows trimmed with tweezers. Medical care of the eyes was provided by medicinal ointments which were known to have been manufactured by the ancient Assyrians.

These people of antiquity rivalled the Egyptians in their liberal use of scent and the production of aromatic substances was one of the most important chemical industries in ancient Mesopotamia. The equipment used to produce aromatics was highly developed and closely resembled the intricate collection of technical implements employed in alchemy. Perfumes and incense were employed for the same purposes as in Egypt, and scent played a vital part in religious ritual, medicine and the manufacturing of cosmetics. Vast quantities of perfumed incense were used in ceremonials and Herodotus states that, at the Temple of Baal in Babylon, '. . . on the greater altar the Chaldeans even offer a thousand talents' weight of frankincense yearly, when they keep the festival of this god'. Scented sesame oil and honey were also used in the embalming of corpses.

Relating to the everyday use of aromatics, the Mesopotamians anointed themselves with sweetened oil extracted from animal fats and vegetable substances, which were perfumed with exotic scents and spices; 'their hair is worn long, and covered with caps, the whole body is perfumed' (Herodotus). Scented oil was also used as a cleansing preparation, for Mesopotamians, like Egyptians, put personal cleanliness high on their list of desirable qualities. Various aromatic plants were also employed as skin cleansers, including tamarisk, the date palm and pine cones. 'May the tamarisk, whereof the tops grow high, cleanse me; may the date palm, which faces every wind, free me; may mastakl plant, which fills the earth, clean me; may the pine cone, which is full of seed corns, free me.' (Akkadian text seventh century BC.) Rue, and potash made from wood ash and soda were other cleansing agents employed in personal hygiene. 'With water I bathed myself. With soda, I cleansed myself. With soda from a shiny basin I purified myself. With the dress of heavenly kingship I clothed myself.' (Sumerian text.) But soap was only used for medicinal purposes and was manufactured from vegetable extracts and oils.

The similarity in their aesthetic attitude to hygiene, combined with their sophisticated use of cosmetics and perfume, allows one to assess collectively the habits of these Middle Eastern civilisations in regard to beauty. There is no doubt that these men and women of antiquity created an atmosphere of mystique around the toilet. Their highly developed use of face paints and perfumery set the example for a beauty routine which was followed throughout the ancient world for centuries to come.

CHAPTER THREE

Cosmetics in Antiquity: Greece and Rome

First she washed all impurity from her desirable person with ambrosia, and anointed herself with rich oil, ambrosial and agreeable, which was odoriferous to her; and the odour of which, when shaken in the brass-founded mansion of Zeus reached even to the earth and to heaven. With this having anointed her body and combed her hair, she arranged with her hands her bright locks, beautiful, ambrosial which flowed from her immortal head (Hera's toilet from the *Iliad* of Homer, translated by C. W. Bateman and R. Mongan)

The ancient Greeks had a more refined approach to cosmetic arts than the early Middle Eastern cultures. The rarified atmosphere of Greece, which encouraged clarity of thought and simple beauty and elegance in the design of architecture and sculpture, contributed to a certain restraint in self-decoration. This refinement is clearly seen in the simplicity of clothing with its sparing use of bright colours and is echoed again in the comparatively light use of cosmetic paints.

The Grecian woman in many cases used no facial make-up, but if she wished to enhance her looks with cosmetics she coloured her cheeks and lips with a vegetable dye made from a root named *polderos* which was similar to alkanet. On the other hand, the Greek courtesans, or *hetaerae*, employed lavish make-up as a mark of their trade in seduction. A bright rouge

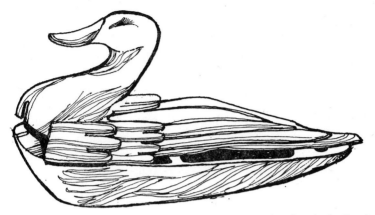

Fig 4 Wooden box for cosmetics in the shape of a swimming duck, Greek or Roman

was applied to their cheeks; their faces were whitened with white lead powder, and their eyes outlined with kohl (*Plate* 6).

A direct comparison in the use of cosmetics by women can be made between the Greeks and the more anciently established civilisation on Crete. The Minoan people, whose culture was in many ways strangely out of context in the Aegean, enjoyed a liberal Middle Eastern attitude to cosmetics and perfumery. Both sexes used oils and aromatics to scent their bodies and on ceremonial occasions adorned themselves with wreaths of sweet scented flowers. Bathrooms were sophisticated in design and lavishly decorated with painted motifs frequently based on marine life. This Minoan talent for decorative art extended to superb frescoes depicting Cretan society. These exquisite small-boned people, with their coiled locks of shining ebony hair, their piquant features and vital sensuality, possessed blanched white skins and large black-rimmed eyes, which in the case of women, and possibly men, indicates their use of kohl and other cosmetic paints.

The reason why Greek women used few cosmetics was possibly due to the masculine orientation of Grecian society.

The Greek man did not wish his wife to be a seductress—he could employ a courtesan for this purpose; he was only concerned with her attributes as a good housewife and mother. Unlike the Egyptian woman, a Grecian lady had little independence and fulfilled a very limited role in society.

The restriction in cosmetic artifice did not, however, extend to the hair. Dyes were frequently employed to change hair colour and these were made from such ingredients as yellow flower petals, potassium solutions and various dye powders. Hair styles emulated the basic simplicity in dress and the women's long tresses were usually swept up on top of the head and fastened with ribbons or metal bands, or contained in a kind of snood (*Plate 7*). However, by the time of Alexander the Great (and after the Roman conquest of Greece), hairstyles had become more elaborate and involved the use of false hair which was frizzed, curled and held in place with a diadem or tiara.

Masculine hairstyles changed with the course of Greek history. In pre-Hellenic times men wore their hair long and were bearded, but by the middle of the fifth century BC it became general to crop hair short and to shave the face. Beards, however, were still worn by old men and in particular philosophers, who used them as a symbol of their freedom from worldly sophistications. Alexander the Great set his seal on the fashion for being clean-shaven, as it was one of the idiosyncrasies of this remarkable soldier to shave his beard even during long and arduous military campaigns.

Shaving the face was an example of the aesthetic attitude to personal hygiene which the ancient Greeks shared with the Middle Eastern cultures. Bathing formed an essential part of the daily toilet and aromatic oils and perfumes were also employed, although these were mainly considered a feminine aid to beauty.

Perfume in ancient Egypt and Mesopotamia had almost

sinister connections with embalming and pagan ceremonial, but the Greeks provided a lighter touch of magic to the mystique of scent. In Greek mythology Aphrodite (Venus) was supposed to have invented perfume and her secret recipe was related to mankind by Aenone, a handmaiden. Helen of Troy was reputed to have emulated Aphrodite in her use of scent and this was offered as one of the reasons for her extraordinary power of attracting men. Legend and myth notwithstanding, Greek women made liberal use of aromatics and the composition of these perfumes is described in the contemporary writings of Theophrastus. Born in 370 BC his principal work involved a detailed classification of Greek plant life, but he also devoted much of his time to writing on aromatics.

> Perfumes are compounded from various parts of the plants: flowers, leaves, twigs, root, wood, fruit and gum; and in most cases the perfume is made from a mixture of several parts. Rose and gilliflower perfumes are made from the flowers: so also is the perfume called Susinon, this too being made from flowers, namely lilies: also the perfumes named from bergamot mint and tufted thyme, kypros, and also the saffron perfume. The crocus which produces this is best in Aegina and Cilicia. Instances of those made from leaves are the perfumes called from myrtle and dropwort: this grows in Cyprus on the hills and is very fragrant: that which grows in Hellas yields no perfume, being scentless . . . from roots are made the perfumes named from iris, spikenard, and sweet marjoram, an ingredient in which is Koston; for it is the root to which this perfume is applied. The Eretrian unguent is made from the root of Kypeiron, which is obtained from Cyclades as well as Enboea. From wood is made what is called 'palm perfume' for they put in what is called the 'spathe', having first dried it. From fruits are made the quince perfume, the myrtle and the bay. The 'Egyptian' is made from several ingredients including cinnamon and myrrh.
>
> (Theophrastus. *Enquiry into Plants* translated by Sir Arthur Hort)

The natural aromatic ingredients for perfumes were manufactured into a finished product through the arts of the perfumer who still relied on an oil base for many of his scents.

41

Theophrastus mentions the use of Egyptian or Syrian 'balanos' oil for this purpose although olive oil was also popular. The 'staying power' of these early perfumes depended in part on the tenacity of the oil but also relied on the strength of the natural scent.

> The lightest are rose-perfume and kypros, which seem to be the best suited to men, as also is lily-perfume. The best for women are myrrh oil, megalion, the Egyptian, sweet marjoram, and spikenard: for these owing to their strength and substantial nature do not easily evaporate and are not easily made to disperse, and a lasting perfume is what women require.
>
> (*Enquiry into Plants*)

The Romans learnt the art of perfumery from the Greek settlements in southern Italy and, through the conquest of Greece, came into contact with other civilised refinements of the toilet. They absorbed Greek ideas on cosmetic care in the same way as, on a higher plane, they absorbed every aspect of Greek culture and made it part of their own way of life.

The growth of the Roman Empire through conquest and subjugation resulted in the establishment of colonies united to Rome by a highly efficient communication system. Extensive imports of foreign goods into the city provided its inhabitants with an enormous range of material amenities, including such luxuries as beauty preparations. Perfumes and unguents were acquired from Egypt and in particular from the famous cosmetic centre of Mendes, whilst the cropped flaxen locks of subjugated Gaulish tribes were imported into Rome to manufacture wigs for wealthy ladies of society.

According to Pliny, the long hair of the Gauls led their country to be nicknamed 'Gallia Comata', or 'Hairy Gaul', and Julius Caesar is reputed to have forced them to cut off their hair as a sign of submission to Roman rule. The truth of this story may be open to doubt, but as blonde wigs were an essential fashion item in ancient Rome the main source of hair was undoubtedly Gaul. The early Christian church made a determined effort to stamp out the fashion for wigs and at this time false flaxen hair was the sign of a prostitute. Roman wigs were never designed to look realistic but were crimped and frizzed with curling irons, after which they were elaborately decorated with ribbons, flowers or ornate jewellery. Natural hair was given the same decorative treatment as wigs and was dressed into a variety of styles. At one stage in Roman history, sculpture portraits of Roman society ladies were executed with detachable hairstyles so that the portrait subject could keep pace with the rapid changes of fashion.

Hair dyes were also in general use by Roman women. They often used recipes for bleaching acquired from the Gauls who made a practice of accentuating their flaxen hair colour by this means. The ingredients for these bleaches included soap compounds of beechwood ash and goat tallow, but unfortunately, as Roman hair did not possess the coarse strength and quality of Germanic locks, bleaching frequently resulted in loss of hair or even baldness. Ovid's plaintive lament to his mistress, Corinna, may well have been echoed by other Roman lovers: 'Did I not say to thee, "Cease to dye thy hair?" And now thou hast no longer any hair to dye. Nevertheless, hadst thou not been stubborn, where was there anything more beautiful than thy hair? . . . Now Germany will send you some slave-girl's hair; a vanquished nation shall furnish thy adornments.' (Ovid. *Ars Amatoria.*) However, fashion prevailed and women continued to employ the use of dyes.

The poor condition of the Roman woman's hair encouraged the creation of 'conditioning' creams to restore tresses to their original beauty. These pomades were made from such ingredients as sheep or bear's grease and marrow extracted from deer bones, whilst extreme remedies included compounds of hellibore and pepper mixed with rat's heads and excrement. The dubious restorative powers of these ointments had little

43

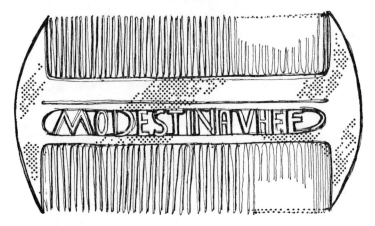

Fig 5 Ivory comb carved with the owner's name, 'Modestina'. No explanation has been offered for the letters 'VHEF', Roman

effect, and clever hairdressing or the use of a wig was needed to disguise diminished locks. The wealthy society lady was provided with this service by her *ornatrix*, a skilled handmaiden who apart from caring for her mistress's hair also presided over the rest of her toilet.

The Roman lady began her day by having her night cream, made from a compound of flour and milk, washed off her face by a slave girl, who would use water scented with perfume essence for this purpose. A goblet of clean water was then brought so that she might rinse her mouth, after which she cleaned her teeth with a toothbrush and dentifrice concocted from powdered horn, pumice stone, or a mixture of burnt potassium or sodium carbonate. Society women who were unable to retain their natural teeth in good condition either employed a dentist to repair the damage with gold, or wore false teeth made from ivory, bone or a cement compound. Next came a bath, and this involved a long period of soaking in perfumed water followed by a massage and rub down with scented oils. Superfluous hair was removed with razors, pumice

44

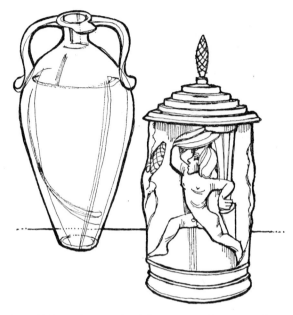

Fig 6 (*left*) rock crystal miniature vase for cosmetics, Roman; (*right*) carved ivory pot for cosmetics, Roman, third century AD

stones or depilatory creams made from medicinal drugs such as bryonia.

After her bath, the Roman lady would have repaired to her boudoir where the *ornatrix* was waiting, with a range of cosmetic paints and implements, to complete the final stage of her mistress's toilet. The dressing table was covered with elegant caskets, boxes, beautifully fashioned cosmetic jars, scissors, files, ivory curry combs, or *stirgilis*, used to remove skin impurities after bathing, and polished copper, silver and even glass hand mirrors, the latter being mounted on lead (*Plate 8*). The *ornatrix* first turned her attention to her mistress's hair which was combed with boxwood, ivory or tortoiseshell combs, crimped with curling irons and dressed into shape.

Then, the face and arms were painted with chalk or white lead powder, whilst lips and cheeks were rouged with a dye made from red ochre or wine dregs. The eyes were accentuated with Egyptian kohl, powdered ash or saffron; lashes were darkened with burnt cork, and eyebrows neatly plucked with tweezers.

The effect of all this cosmetic elaboration was frequently overstated and many Romans criticised women for their excessive use of artifice: 'Artifice is a fine thing when it's not perceived' and 'the art that adorns you should be unsuspected. Who but would feel a sensation of disgust if the paint on your face were so thick that it oozed down on your breasts?' (Ovid. *Ars Amatoria*.) For this reason Ovid warned Roman lovers that an unexpected visit to their mistresses' boudoirs might upset

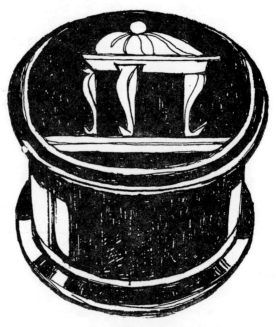

Fig 7 Clay rouge pot discovered at Naucratis still containing traces of rouge, fourth century BC

46

their image of natural feminine beauty. 'You'll find she's got boxes containing concoctions of all colours of the rainbow, and you'll see the paint trickling down in warm streams on to her breasts. The whole place stinks like Phineus' dinner-table, and I've often felt as if I was going to be sick.' (*Ars Amatoria*.)

Roman men, however, themselves used a large range of cosmetic preparations and many of these concotions were employed by the barber, or *tonsor*, as part of his after-shave treatment. The Roman who did not possess a skilled servant to shave his beard started the day with a visit to the barber's shop, and in some cases this system was preferred as these establishments were great centres for gossip. The *tonsor* required considerable skill, as the Roman razor, or *novacula*, was made of iron which quickly corroded, became blunt and as a result cut and gashed the face. To repair the damage, plasters made from spiders' webs soaked in oil and vinegar were applied and perfumed ointments were used to soothe the skin. Blemishes were also disguised by small 'patches' of material known as *splenia lunata*. As an alternative to shaving, there were depilatories made from such ingredients as resin, pitch, white vine or ivy gum extracts, ass's fat, she-goat's gall, bat's blood and powdered viper. If these drastic remedies proved ineffective, many men followed the example of Julius Caesar who had his facial hairs individually plucked out with tweezers.

Scipio Africanus had set the mode for being clean-shaven; no doubt his fame as the conqueror of Hannibal led to this fashion being generally adopted. The first shave of a youth came to be regarded as the arrival of masculine adulthood and was offered as a token to his favourite god. Perhaps because of this connection with masculinity, the clean-shaven look persisted until the reign of the Emperor Hadrian who grew a beard, reputedly to hide a bad skin, after which this fashion was followed by many Romans.

Hadrian and Nero, during their separate reigns, set a vogue

for artificially curled hairstyles for men, although these were mainly popular with dandies who also dyed and scented their hair with cassia and cinnamon perfumes. A general trend in male vanity, however, encouraged the fashion for wigs, as many Romans became prematurely bald and required a disguise for this defect. Caligula is supposed to have worn a wig to hide his identity whilst prowling around the brothels of ancient Rome, and Caracalla wore a blonde wig to ingratiate himself with Germanic tribesmen during a visit to their settlement.

Another aspect of the male toilet which was of prime importance to the Roman man, for social as well as cosmetic reasons, was his daily sojourn to the baths of the city. These were equipped with gymnasia, libraries and beautiful gardens in addition to the ornately decorated marble baths. There was a cold room, *frigidarium*; warm room, *tepidarium*; and hot room, *calidarium*, which operated on the Turkish principle of hot water and steam baths; and an extra hot room, *laconicum*, for medicinal treatments. Private villas contained their own superb baths:

> From thence you enter into the grand and spacious cooling-room belonging to the baths, from the opposite walls of which two curved basins are thrown out, so to speak; these are large enough, if you consider that the sea is close by. Contiguous to this is the anointing-room, then the sweating room and beyond that the furnace; adjoining are two other little bathing-rooms which are fitted up in an elegant rather than costly manner. (The epistles of Pliny translated by William Melmoth)

The sheer luxury of life in ancient Rome with its emphasis on comfort and leisure and its enjoyment of beauty and fashion, is reflected in the ritual of the toilet. Both sexes devoted several hours a day to the care of their bodies and the embellishment of their faces by cosmetic means. Roman ingenuity in design was evident in the manufacture of every form of toilet implement: the standard of perfection attained in major works of

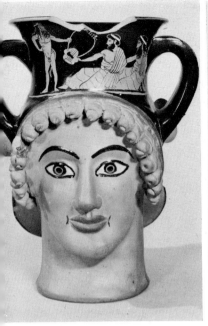

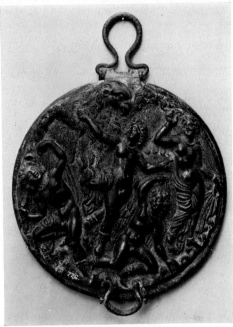

(*above left*) Moulded head vase. Greek, *c* 470 BC. Greek courtesans would have painted their ~~f~~ in the fashion illustrated on this unusual vase. Kohl and lip rouge were also commonly ~~used~~ by Roman society ladies.

(*below*) Clay drinking cup. Greek, 490–80 BC. Greek styles of hairdressing are illustrated ~~on th~~ese figures; the one seated has elaborately curled ringlets.

(*above right*) Bronze folding mirror. Etruscan, 200 BC. A fine example of the type of beauti~~fully~~ worked toilet implement used in ancient Rome.

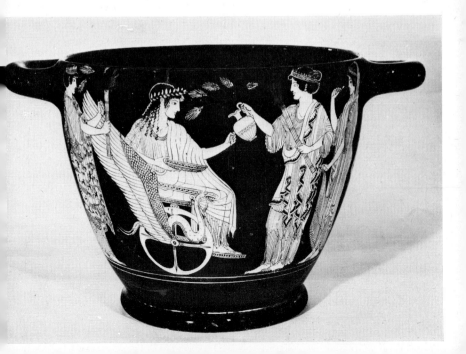

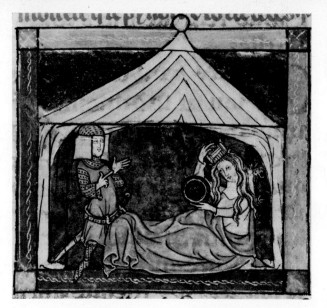

9 (left) A lady at her toilet. Fourteenth centur The double-sided comb is similar to the one illustrated in Fig 9 (p 61

10 (right) Medieval perfumer's shop. On the counter, the mirrors are illustrated with faces to simulate reflections.

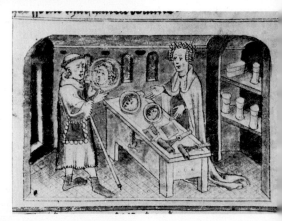

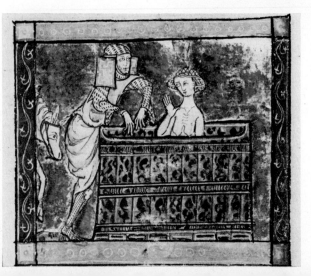

11 (left) A lady bathing. Public bath-houses simil to those of ancient Rom were re-introduced to England after the Crusa Individual baths were al taken, often involving a eccentric assortment of apparatus (see quotatio from the Boke of Nurtur pp 62–3).

art is seen again in beautifully fashioned boxes, caskets and other cosmetic containers. In their attitude to hygiene and their use of perfumery and beauty preparations, the Romans set a standard of civilised elegance which can scarcely be rivalled by any other culture.

PART TWO

A History of Cosmetics in England

CHAPTER FOUR

Early Britain and the Middle Ages

Faire is lady in hire bour;
And so is knyght in his armure
(Attributed to Adam Davie. 'The Marchal of Stratford atte Bowe',
King Alisaunder)

The sophistication of the great Middle Eastern and Mediter-ranean cultures, with their eminently refined approach to living and highly developed appreciation of art and beauty, found no parallel in the wildly rugged island of Britain which at a later period in history was still isolated from the worldly influences of these civilisations.

The grey windswept hills and thick forests haunted by wolves and wild boar offered little potential accommodation for humans and the inclement weather was a constant barrier to human comfort. The Celtic nomads who had settled on the island were as savage and wildlooking as the land which they chose to inhabit. They were clad in animal skins and their thick long hair was dyed red in a mixture of water boiled with lime, whilst their bodies were patterned with painted designs. The word Pict comes from *Picti*, meaning 'painted', and was an apt description of people who covered themselves in coloured images of birds and animals. This habit had little to do with 'cosmetic' embellishment, but was a means of establishing a

53

tribal identity and, within the tribal unit, of distinguishing social rank. A chieftain might paint himself with large elaborate designs whereas men of a humbler social order had to be content with a small single motif. During the Roman occupation, when the ancient Britons adopted conventional clothes, they transferred the painted designs of birds and animals from their bodies to their shields, and eventually these images formed the basis for heraldic devices.

Although the wild appearance of the ancient Britons might have indicated otherwise, a developed form of social organisation and culture existed before the Roman conquest. The Druids, despite their reputation for witchcraft and paganism, had a controlling and civilising influence on the Celtic people and were renowned for their prowess in primitive medicine. Through their skill with herbs, they concocted the closest parallel to cosmetics at this period in the form of herbal ointments, which they reputedly imbued with magical powers to cure wounds or enhance beauty. Perfume, as such, was unknown in pre-Roman Britain, but the Druids were not insensible to the beauty of fragrance and employed the use of aromatic herbs. On ceremonial occasions, Druidesses wreathed their heads in crowns of verbena which apart from its sweet scent was a particularly magical plant according to Druid herbal lore.

During the several hundred years of Britain's colonisation by Rome the aspect of the island and its people changed radically. The untamed country was cultivated, roads were constructed and towns were built. The dark and mystic Celtic culture was replaced by a highly developed and complex civilisation which offered comfort, and even luxury. The Celts adopted an approximation of Roman dress and, at a more sophisticated level, the cosmetics and perfumes of their conquerors.

The departure of the Romans in AD 429 had little immediate

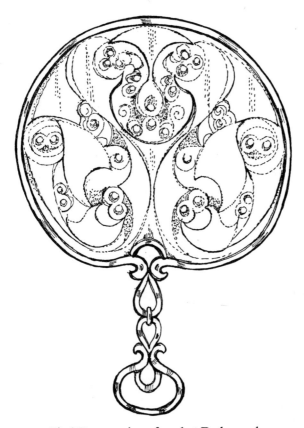

Fig 8 Bronze mirror found at Desborough,
Northamptonshire, first century AD

effect on the Briton's way of life which remained essentially
Roman, but during the course of time the island was subjected
to repeated invasions by barbaric Teutonic tribes. Then,
although the Roman influence remained strong, invasions by
Angles, Saxons and Jutes over a long period gradually changed
the existing culture. These German tribes reintroduced body
painting to Britain, covering themselves in blue 'woad' tattooed

55

designs and, like the Celts before the Roman Conquest, they dyed their long hair red or bleached it to a paler shade of flaxen blonde.

The Nordic invaders made a particular fetish of their hair. Men cultivated luxuriant beards and both sexes wore their hair long. Much time and attention was devoted to grooming it to their satisfaction, and the elaborate combs and pins found in Teutonic tombs are evidence of the interest in this aspect of their appearance. The Danes were renowned for their exceptional wealth of hair, and the male courtiers of King Canute were reputed to have waist-length hair which they groomed and combed at least once every day.

The Teutonic influence erased many of the refinements enjoyed by the Romanised Briton. To these changes the early Christian church made its contribution. The Christian missionaries declared that bathing was an evil, ungodly vanity and thus the newly Christian Britons rejected the Roman custom of taking baths. Early Christians who wore wigs were even excommunicated by the church for this attempt at self-improvement.

The cosmetics and perfumes of Roman Britain had also disappeared and contemporary records illustrate a return to herbal potions and ointments which were used in lieu of cosmetic preparations:

> For an eye salve, take aloes and zedoary, laurel berries and pepper, shave them small, and lay fresh cow's butter in water, then take a broad whetstone and rub the butter on the whetstone with copper so that it may be pretty rough, then add some part of the worts thereto, then put the paste into a brass vessel, let it stand for nine days, and let some one turn it every day; afterwards melt it in the same brass vessel, strain it through a cloth, afterwards put it into whatever vessel thou wilt, use it when need be. This salve is good for infirmity of every sort which aileth the eyes. (*Leechdoms, Wortcunning and Starcraft*. A collection of Anglo-Saxon documents edited by Rev Oswald Cockayne)

Due to a rough, out of doors life the Anglo-Saxons appear to have suffered greatly from chapped hands as there are numerous 'hand creams' to be found among contemporary recipes:

To Protect Peeling or Sore Hands

Take a hand full of beet and a hand full of lettuce and a hand full of coriander, and pound all together; then take crumbs, and put them into water, and the worts with them, and then warm the worts well in the water and the crumbs with it; then work up a poultice thereof and bind upon the hands for one night, and do this as long as need may be (*Leechdoms, Wortcunning and Starcraft*)

Yet another 'hand cream' includes lily of the valley as an ingredient: 'For sore of hands, take this same wort Apollinaris, pound it with old lard without salt, add thereto a cup of old wine, and let that be heated without smoke, and of the lard let there be by weight of one pound; pound together in the manner which thou mightest work a plaister, and lay to the hand.' (*Leechdoms, Wortcunning and Starcraft.*) Apart from their soothing and healing properties, the Saxons believed, as the Druids had before them, that herbs contained magical powers. Individual plants were used for particular purposes; thus lily of the valley was good for the hands and foxgloves or mint were used in recipes to purge the skin of spots.

These Saxon recipes are the only example of 'cosmetic' care at this period, but there is evidence of perfume being introduced to Britain during the reign of King Ethelstan. The king's sister was courted by Hugh, King of the Franks, and his ambassador brings amongst other gifts for the Saxon princess 'perfumes such as never had been seen in England before'. (*Chronicles of William of Malmesbury.*)

In 1066 William of Normandy invaded England and defeated Harold, the Saxon king, at Hastings. The Saxon spies sent out before the battle to assess the enemy's strength are reputed to have returned with reports of having seen an army of 'priests' and not soldiers. This misconception arose from the fact that the Normans were all clean shaven and their hair was shaved off from the back of the head in an exaggerated 'short back and sides' style which gave them a monk-like appearance. It is strange that Harold's spies were misled by a cropped hair cut as, according to William of Malmesbury's description, the Saxons also favoured a shorter hairstyle at this period: 'The English at that time wore short garments reaching to the mid-knee; they had their hair cropped, their beards shaven, their arms laden with golden bracelets, their skin adorned with punctured designs'.

The Norman influence in England added refinement to the Saxon way of life. Norman French manners, customs and fashions had been previously introduced to the English court during the reign of Edward the Confessor, but after the Norman conquest the French style of living was more generally adopted by the Saxon nobility. The contemporary English appearance was also affected by the Norman influence. The 'priest's' hairstyle became fashionable with the Saxon aristocracy and the barbaric habit of tattooing the body less common. Cosmetics were obviously not among the innovations introduced by the invaders since, after the conquest, Saxon women's faces remained as untouched as ever by artificial colouring.

The Englishwoman's vanity was denied any scope whatsoever by the new Norman fashion for concealing feminine tresses under a kerchief. The Saxon matron, according to Teutonic custom, had taken a particular pride in displaying her long, braided hair, but now only young girls were permitted to continue with this tradition. However, during the reign of Henry I, his Saxon queen, Matilda, revived the old Germanic fashion by allowing her hair to remain flowing and loose. Men, it seems, were encouraged by this feminine example and also grew their hair long. 'They vied with women in length of locks, and wherever they were defective, put on false tresses, forgetful, or rather ignorant, of the saying of the apostle, if a man nurtures his hair it is a shame on him.' (*Chronicles of William of Malmesbury*.) The early twelfth-century man's use of false locks to supplement his own hair illustrates the importance of this aspect of his toilet. Handsome forked beards, somewhat Assyrian in style, were also fashionable at this time; these were groomed into shape and dressed with wax.

The attitude of ecclesiastics, judging from William of Malmesbury's condemnation of male vanity, was totally against any form of adornment or self-decoration; it is ironical, therefore, that a movement inspired by contemporary religious ideals should have been responsible for the introduction of cosmetics to Europe. The Crusades, which introduced European men to the luxuries of Middle Eastern life, had a profound effect on the dress, toilet and customs of the Middle Ages. European men were inspired to leave their own countries on a quest which owed as much to a desire for change and the excitement of battle as to religious or spiritual involvement. Mixed motives were also responsible for the women's crusade led by Eleanor of Aquitaine, wife of King Louis of France. Aristocratic Frenchwomen, it seems, were unwilling to allow their husbands to abandon them to a long period of chastity, and promises of infidelity on their part threatened to disrupt a crusade led by the French king. Queen Eleanor, who later divorced Louis and married Henry II of England, decided to organise these female rebels into a women's army. Wearing crusader uniforms, they would follow the men on their spiritual journey offering them the comforts of home life during the crusade. The Church frowned on this feminine escapade, and with good reason, for the noblewomen's example encouraged a motley selection of female camp followers to join the Crusades. Religious men believed that these women were largely responsible for the degeneration of the Second Crusade as reports

reached Europe of gay orgies round camp fires, where trouba-
dours abandoned their lyrical serenades for bawdy alehouse
songs, and of European women covering their faces with
Eastern cosmetics before a battle so that they would attract the
Saracens should the crusaders suffer defeat.

The medieval Church's lack of confidence in female morality
may have resulted in an exaggeration of these stories regarding
the use of cosmetics by camp followers, but it is a fact that
Eastern cosmetic materials and toilet articles were introduced
to European crusaders during their time in the Middle East.
The contemporary eyewitness reports of the Crusades record
the overwhelming impression that Eastern luxuries made on
the crusading knight. Apart from acquiring his share of the
priceless booty from ambushed Turkish and Saracen caravans,
the crusader also developed a taste for the comparatively easy
luxury of Eastern living. It is therefore hardly surprising that
the crusaders brought back many commodities and customs
which had delighted them in the Holy Land (*Plate 9*).

Apart from cosmetic preparations, the crusaders returned
home with aromatics and perfumes (*Plate 10*). During the later
Crusades, Richard I, son of Henry II and Eleanor of Aquitaine,
had conquered Cyprus, and the perfume 'Eau de Chypre',
which takes its name from the island, was introduced to
Europe at this period. In the fourteenth century *oyselets de
chypre* were made from a mixture compounded into a paste
and shaped like little birds, which were then burnt to allow
the aroma of scent to escape and sweeten the air. Crusaders
also returned to Europe with the recipe for rose-water and
introduced the Eastern custom of offering bowls of rose-
water to guests after a banquet. Entranced by the sweetly
scented flowers they had seen in the Middle East, the crusaders
brought home many of these floral plants, including the lily
which became one of the emblems of romantic chivalry.
English knights also introduced to England the Saracen bride's

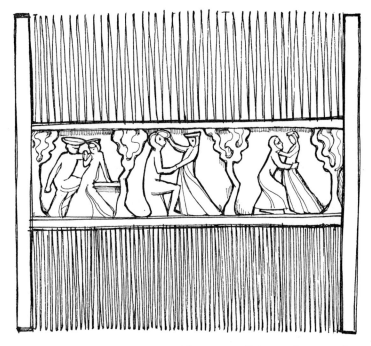

Fig 9 Ivory comb engraved with scenes of lovers in a garden, French, fourteenth century

custom of wearing an orange blossom wreath on her wedding day.

The Eastern influence became apparent in costume and hairstyles. Men wore turban-shaped hats and elaborate hoods, whilst their hair was cut short in the fashion adopted during the Crusades when long hairstyles had proved impractical in the hot climate of the Holy Land. Women's headdresses became ornate and the Eastern love of extravagance seems to have continued as an influence in female headgear during the course of the Middle Ages. Styles varied from a simple veil or wimple to vast edifices resembling towers, winged birds and

61

butterflies. Although women's hair during the late Middle Ages was usually hidden under a headdress, it made an occasional appearance in ornate gold hair nets known as 'crespines' and gilded latticework pads described as 'templars'. Tubes of silk entwined with gold cord bound long plaits which were supplemented with false hair to extend their length to below the waist.

English crusaders re-introduced bathing to England and public baths similar to those of ancient Rome were built in many large towns. The knights had no doubt enjoyed the Middle Eastern style of bathing in the Holy Land and the design of medieval bath-houses copied the basic principles of a Turkish bath, with special sweating rooms and hot water or steam baths which were produced by dropping heated stones into water. Bathing was mixed, a fact which must have displeased contemporary churchmen. It is unlikely that the public baths were used on any regular basis; cleanliness was probably a secondary consideration compared with the therapeutic effects of heat and warmth in a cold climate, and the additional attraction of massage facilities which were provided by some bath-houses. English lords, who preferred bathing in the privacy of their castles or manor houses, trained their 'chamberlains' to prepare a bath; from contemporary description, this combined an Eastern use of aromatics with an attempt at re-creating the comfort and luxury enjoyed by the crusaders when in the East (*Plate 11*). The 'bathroom' was hung with sheets containing aromatic herbs and sweet-scented flowers; and sponges, placed on the floor, were covered by another sheet. The lord could then sit in cushioned comfort whilst his 'chamberlain' or squire rinsed him down with perfumed water.

Hang shetis round about the rooff; do thus as y meene, every shete full of flowres and herbis soote and grene, and looke ye have sponges v or vj theron to sytte or lene:

A basyn full in youre hand of herbis hote and fresche, and with a soft sponge in hand, his body that ye wasche, Rynse hym with rose water warme and feire uppon hym flasche.

(The Duties of a Chamberlain included in the
Boke of Nurture by John Russell, usher and Marshal
to Humphrey, Duke of Gloucester. Early fifteenth century)

This recipe illustrates the emphasis on therapy as opposed to cleanliness and there is little doubt that this was the main reason for bathing.

Apart from the influence on fashions and toilet, the Crusades had introduced to European knights the Saracen tradition of chivalry which was highly developed at this period. Moorish warriors were trained to observe exacting standards of behaviour in war or love, and their mode of conduct in either situation was governed by set rules and principles. Their lyrical minstrelsy of war and love, formal courtesy to ladies and ritual etiquette were echoed in European romantic chivalry which exerted its influence in England from the thirteenth century until the end of the Middle Ages.

The chivalric attitude to love based on high romance and courtly ritual put women on a pedestal, which contrasted strangely with their actual status in medieval society. A woman was a mere pawn used in marriage to gain power in some political manoeuvre or to acquire property should she belong to a wealthy family. The medieval view of female beauty was restricted by women's social status and by a stereotyped idea of feminine perfection, as idealised in chivalric love poetry. Female looks were standardised into a pale fair-haired prettiness with no hint of individuality in character or appearance to disturb its wan image (*Plate 12*).

One bizarre fashion which contributed to this uniformity of facial beauty was that women, using tweezers, plucked all the hair from their eyebrows, temples and necks (*Plate 13*). The

63

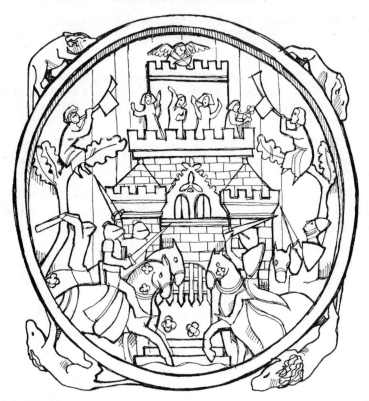

Fig 10 Ivory mirror case, the carving shows the storming of the Castle of Love, German, *c* 1350–60

obvious excuse for this masochistic practice was to draw attention to the elaborate headdresses worn at the time. The true reason, however, was probably the desire to eliminate any idiosyncratic faults and to simulate the perfect elongated oval face which accorded with the contemporary ideal image.

The model medieval female face was always represented as having small neat features and pale grey eyes. The complexion was usually compared to the waxen whiteness of a lily enhanced by rose-red tints on cheeks and lips, whilst the hair was fre-

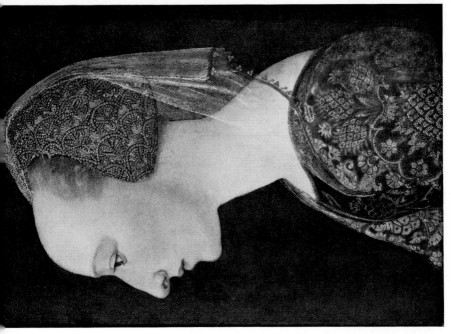

Rogier Van der Weyden. A medieval ideal of beauty as admired in England. The face is robbed of any individual idiosyncrasy by the contemporary fashion for plucking all hair from the forehead and eyebrows. The pale complexion was another common feature of medieval women's looks.

13 (*right*) Portrait of a lady in red. Florentine school. An extreme example of hair plucking which gives the impression of baldness.

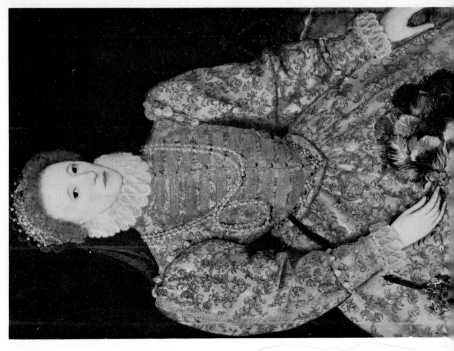

14 (*left*) Portrait of Anne Boleyn by an unknown artist. The Tudor ideal of beauty has her hair drawn back under the pearled archway of a headdress which frames her white oval face. Her eyes have the secretive expression of Leonardo da Vinci's 'Mona Lisa'.

15 (*right*) Queen Elizabeth I by an unknown artist. Her brows and forehead were plucked. Her pale complexion was emphasised by the application of white lead powder, afterwards glazed with egg-white

quently likened to spun gold. An excellent description of medieval beauty appears in Chaucer's version of *The Romaunt of the Rose*:

> Hir heer was as yelowe of hewe
> As any basin scoured newe.
> Hir flesh as tendre as is chike, [chicken]
> With bente browes, smothe and slike;
> And by mesure large were
> the opening of hir yen [eyes] clere.
> Hir nose of good proporcionn,
> Hir yën greye as a faucoun [falcon]
> With swete breeth and wel savoured,
> Hir face whyt and wel coloured,
> With litel mouth, and round to see;
> A clove chin eek hadde she.

Another passage in this poem deals in lyrical terms with the complexion:

> Hir flesh was tendre as dewe of flour [flower]
> Hir chere [appearance] was simple as byrde in bour;
> As whyt as lilie or rose in rys
> Hir face, gentil and tretys [graceful].

It is an interesting fact that the emblems of romantic chivalry, the rose and lily, set the colour for complexions for a period of several centuries. During the Middle Ages a white skin was an essential feature of perfect beauty and the winged veiling of contemporary headdresses served a useful purpose in protecting complexions from sunburn. For the same reason, gloves were always worn when out of doors.

> And for to kepe hir hondes faire
> Of gloves whyte she hadde a paire
> (*The Romaunt of the Rose*)

Protection from the sun was one way to keep complexions pale and fair, but there is evidence in France that make-up was also used to enhance naturally white skin tones. The Crusades had introduced Eastern cosmetics to the Continent, and French sources mention the use of powder, rouge, hair colourants and a variety of toilet implements, such as ear-pickers, toothpicks and even tongue-scrapers. Apart from more elaborate cosmetic ingredients, French beauty preparations contained basic natural materials. Wheat powder, or *blaunchet*, was used to blanch the face; hair was washed in 'lye', a mixture of wood ash and water, and wine was incorporated into hair dyes. Bleaches were also used by Frenchwomen to lighten their hair to a fashionable saffron yellow.

There is little contemporary evidence of the employment of these items of toiletry in England, but it can be reasonably supposed that some English noblewomen followed the example of French court ladies, for although France and England were alienated by the Hundred Years War the English court was still influenced by French fashions and customs. However, the comparatively scanty information available would indicate that English ladies on the whole employed fewer cosmetics than their French counterparts.

Cosmetic materials were certainly available to Englishwomen of the Middle Ages, as the Crusades had encouraged trade with the East and the combined Guild of Pepperers and Spicers, known as the Fraternity of St Anthony, imported quantities of Arabian aromatic spices, oils, gum resins and perfumed essences. The manufacture of these raw materials into facial cosmetics would also have been possible at this period, as the Arab science of alchemy had many followers in England and English alchemists already treated the creation of perfumes as their special preserve. Thomas Norton's *Ordinall of Alchemy* makes a particular reference to scent:

Pleasant odours ingendered be shall
Of Cleane and Pure substance and fumigale,
As it appeareth in Amber, Warde and Mirrhe,
Good for a Woman, Such things pleaseth her.

66

While it appears that little use was made of the alchemists' potential talent in the field of cosmetics, once the store of Eastern toilet preparations brought home by crusader husbands had been exhausted, the Englishwoman could rely on cosmetics imported from the Continent or on home-made recipes for beauty no doubt based on the herbal remedies of the Saxon period.

Since availability was not the problem, it is reasonable to assume that it was the attitude of the puritan element in the medieval church that restrained Englishwomen from using cosmetics. Ecclesiastical puritans totally condemned artificial vanities as the devil's evil influence on womankind. Aristocratic French ladies may have partially ignored priestly tirades against fashionable artifice, but Englishwomen accustomed to the slightly less worldly environment of the English court were more likely to have been deeply affected by the Church's condemnation. The Church wielded immense power over medieval society and it is impossible to overemphasise the effect of religious teachings on the contemporary mind. The Church demanded absolute unity of belief in its narrow and literal interpretation of the Bible, and this faith in the factual substance of biblical texts led ecclesiastics to interpret as literal truth the idea that man was fashioned in God's image. The Church for this reason believed that the use of cosmetics tampered with man's, and therefore God's, image which was the most evil of sins.

This puritan ecclesiastical attitude was upheld by many contemporary men and in Chaucer's version of *The Romaunt of the Rose* he personifies 'Beautee' as a woman who uses no 'peynte' and who leaves her brows unplucked. However, the best written example of contemporary puritanism regarding cosmetics and vanity is provided in *The Book of the Knight of La Tour Landry*, which was translated from the French during the reign of Henry VI. Geoffrey de la Tour Landry wrote his book as a moral guide for his three motherless daughters. It incorporates both contemporary religious and secular puritan attitudes to vanity, emphasising the medieval belief that make-up destroyed God's image in womankind:

> Whi sufficithe it not that God hathe formed man and woman after hys owne shape, in the whiche the aungeles so moche delitithe hem, for ioye to see God in the visage? For, and God wolde, hym nedithe not to have made hem women, but dome bestis or serpentis. Alas! whi take women none hede of the gret love that God hathe yene hem, to make hem after his figure?

The stories which make up the book all have a moral message against the use of artifice and list the appalling punishments that await vain women:

> Ther was a ladi that duelled fast bi the chirche, that toke every day so longe tyme to make redy that it made weri and angri the person of the chirche and parissheres to abide after her . . . And as God wolde shew for ensaumple, atte the same tyme and houre as she loked in a mirrour, in stede of the mirrour, the develle turned to her his ars, the whiche was so foule and orible that for ferde [fear] she was sike longe; and atte the laste God sent her her witte and she was chastised, and wolde no more make folke to mouse after her, but wold be sonner arraied and atte the chirche thanne ani other—And therfor, daughtres, takithe here your myrrour and ensaumple to live alle such lewde folyes and counterfeting, poppinge [tricking out] and peintinge.

Men were also warned against the evil qualities of vain women and taking an interest in their own masculine vanity. *The Boke of Knyghthode,* translated by Stephen Scrope during the fifteenth century from an earlier French version written by Christine de Pisan, provided men with a guide to the virtuous ways of a true knight. To achieve the high standard of perfection expected of him, the aspiring knight had to pass a series of moral tests. One classical story is retold in medieval terms in *The Boke of Knyghthode:*

And thanne Paris gaff his sentence and forsoke bothe knyghthode, wisdom and riches for Venus, to whom he gaff the appyll; for the whiche after that Troye was dystryd. This is to understonde, because that Paris was not chevallrous ne reche, he sette be noo thing, but all his thought was on love, and therfor gaffe he the appill to Venus. Wherefor it is seide to the goode knyght that he should not demene hym so.

Venus represented to the contemporary mind the ultimate in idle vanity, and this sensual goddess was the opposite of the medieval ideal of womankind whose cool beauty and pious nature were praised in poems on courtly love. The examples of *The Book of the Knight of La Tour Landry* and *The Boke of Knyghthode* are evidence of the contemporary rejection of cosmetic artifice and vanity.

The rigidly controlled way of life dictated by the Church, with its repressive moral attitudes, restrained free artistic expression and imaginative thinking. Although magnificent works of architecture, lyrical poetry, beautiful needlework and extraordinary fashions contrive to create a nostalgically beguiling picture of the Middle Ages, a degree of conformity permeates medieval artistic creation giving this picture the static quality of a carefully worked tapestry. Chaucer's *Canterbury Tales* with its appreciation of human character and fallibility seems out of keeping in an age when human weaknesses, such as vanity, were considered totally vicious and individual beauty was robbed of its essential character by art. The use of cosmetics, which depends on a sympathetic understanding of human vanity and an interest in facial beauty, had little hope of general acceptance until the end of the fifteenth century when the rigidly set conventions of medieval life were disrupted by the Renaissance.

CHAPTER FIVE

Late Fifteenth and Sixteenth Centuries

Her haire fine threads of finest gold,
In curled knots man's thought to hold,
But that her fore-head sayes, In me
A Whiter beautie you may see;
Whiter!—in deede more white than snow
Which on cold winter's face doth grow.
(Sir Philip Sidney. *Arcadia*)

The Renaissance in Italy marked the end of the Middle Ages in Europe. The human spirit so long confined by the restrictive pattern of medieval life poured out in a wealth of artistic expression. Inspired by the Hellenic age, Renaissance man abandoned himself to the new freedom of intellectual invention. Romantic love and the crude strength of the Middle Ages were refined into a more sympathetic appreciation of all that is exquisite in the human form and all that is exciting in a liberated imagination. The ideal man of the late fifteenth and sixteenth centuries combined all facets of human endeavour. He was a poet, artist, scholar and adventurer, most aptly described as 'A Man for all Seasons'. It is perhaps scarcely surprising that, in an age when the European intellect turned in upon the nature of man as an emancipation from old constraints upon the imagination, there developed a new style in personal appearance and adornment.

In England, the spirit of the Renaissance was slow to awaken and only came to full fruition in the reign of Elizabeth I. However, the fashions of the early Tudor period illustrate the influence of Italy. A Tudor gentleman most particularly represents the Renaissance element in England with his richly coloured clothes, padded out to vast proportions to exaggerate his masculine form and to give an impression of powerful, latent virility. But the Tudor woman still retains the rigid immobility of a Gothic carving with her dresses of weighty fabric embossed with lavish embroidery. The inflexibility of her garments give her a static splendour so admirably illustrated in Holbein's portraits.

Holbein's detailed paintings of his contemporary subject give a clear picture of the Tudor ideal of beauty. Henry VIII epitomises an ideal of masculine handsomeness with his pale complexion, light red-gold hair and beard set off to advantage by gargantuan expanses of warm-textured velvet and the glowing light and shade of embroidered silk. Tudor feminine beauty is perfectly represented in a portrait of Anne Boleyn by an unknown artist of the day (*Plate 14*). Her hair is drawn smoothly back under the pearled archway of a Tudor headdress, which frames her white oval face and draws attention to her dark eyes with their secretive expression reminiscent of Leonardo da Vinci's 'Mona Lisa'.

For both sexes a pale complexion remained, as in the Middle Ages, a desired feature of their appearance. A light white powder and blush of rouge may have been used by a few women to enhance their complexions, but cosmetics were not generally used until Elizabeth's reign. Instead, preventive measures were taken to ensure the preservation of a white skin. Undoubtedly, the Tudor gable headdress, which owed its inspiration to the architectural conventions of the day, sheltered the face from the sun and, later in the century, the same purpose was served by the 'French hood' which shaded the forehead.

71

Although cosmetics were not much used in the early Tudor period, perfume was popular with both sexes. Scents were imported from the Continent, but men and women also created their own recipes chiefly based on herbal properties. Henry VIII was reputed to have invented this recipe: 'Of compound water take six spoonfuls, as much of Rose-Water, a quarter of an ounce of fine sugar, two grains of Musk, two grains of Amber-greece, two of Civet: boyl it softly together: all the house will smell of Cloves'. (Sir Hugh Platt, *Delightes for Ladies*, 1602.) Perfume was an aesthetic necessity in Tudor and Elizabethan times, acting as a deodorant. An additional 'deodorant' was provided by the pomander.

Pomanders (*pommes d'ambre*, literally 'amber apples') were introduced to England about 1500. The 'apple', which was frequently attached to the sash ends of a girdle, contained scents and herbs, including nutmeg, rosewater, aloes and ambergris. One Elizabethan recipe is more detailed:

> Of Beazon take one dram and a half, of Storax half a dram, of Lignum Aloes in fine powder half a scruple, of Labanum half an ounce: powder all these very fine, and fearce them thorow lawn: and then take of Musk a dram, Amber-greece ten grains, Civet ten grains, and dissolve them in a hot Morter with a little rosewater, and so make them them into a Pomander, putting into it six grains of Civet. (Sir Hugh Platt. *Delightes for Ladies.*)

Pomanders continued to be fashionable throughout the reign of Elizabeth I. Apart from their aromatic quality, men and women believed in their medicinal value. Presumably they felt that no disease could flourish in the proximity of such a delightful scent.

Elizabeth's coronation on 15 January 1559 marked the beginning of a new phase of the Renaissance in England. The young queen epitomised the spirit of the age, combining scholarship, statecraft and queenly authority with feminine

72

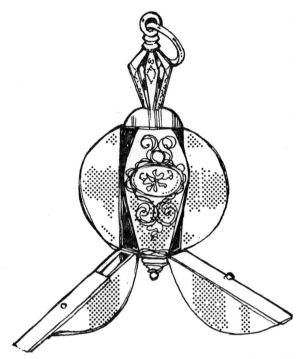

Fig 11 Pomander or scent case in gilt set with small enamels, Dutch, *c* 1600

allure. She attracted to her court brilliant and unusual men who in every way reflected a new mode of thought. The Gothic shadow of early Tudor England ebbed away before the promise of a new and brilliant future. The fashions of the day reflected this change in attitude. The ponderous magnificence of early Tudor costume disappeared in favour of lighter padded clothes, which made use of lavish and bright coloured fabrics, exquisite embroidery and huge lace ruffs. An amalgam of these features gave fashions a feminine quality.

This was certainly due to Elizabeth. It would be true to say that no single individual has ever exerted such an influence

73

on the fashions and beauty of a period. The large ruff characteristic of this era was adapted by Elizabeth from an earlier Spanish version, and the fine filigree of white lace made a perfect foil for her pale complexion and elaborately curled red-gold hair. In the queen was personified the Elizabethan ideal of beauty (*Plate 15*).

A Mayden Queen that shone as Titan's Ray
In glistring gold and perelesse pretious stone
(Spenser. 'The Faerie Queene')

When she ascended the throne at twenty-five years of age her natural handsomeness was beyond dispute, but the preservation of her beauty became an obsession stemming from feminine vanity and perhaps a sense of insecurity which was both political and emotional. Certainly this interest in preserving her appearance prompted Elizabeth to resort to the use of ingenious cosmetic artifice.

Cosmetics had begun to be generally used by the year of her coronation. The main inspiration for their use as an aid to beauty came from Italy, where the women were well in advance of their English contemporaries. Foreign ambassadors commented favourably on the natural complexions of Englishwomen in comparison to the heavily painted faces of Italians. In Italy, women used cosmetics liberally, employing a range of tints to colour their eyelids and even their teeth. The influence of the ancient Hellenic culture that inspired the Renaissance is illustrated in the preference for dyed blonde hair or saffron wigs dressed and curled into a contemporary adaptation of an ancient Greek hairstyle. Catholic priests were severely critical of this use of artifice, but the mood of the Renaissance prevailed over these dictates and Italians continued to dress lavishly and adorn their faces with cosmetics. Many contemporary laymen, too, felt that the use of 'paint', as cosmetics

74

were aptly named, had reached an excess. Even such sophisticated men as Count Baldassare Castiglione were disgusted with the sight of painted women at the Italian court:

> All women generally have a great desire to be, and when they canne not be, at the least to appear beautyfall. Therefore where nature in some part hath not done her devoyr therein, they endeavour themselves to supply it with out. Of this ariseth the trymming of the face, with such studye and many times peines, the pilling of the browes and forehead, and the usynge of all these maner wayes and the abydyng of such lothsomenesse as you women believe are kepte very secrete from men, and yet do all men know them (Count Baldassare Castiglione. *The Book of the Courtier*. Translated by Sir Thomas Hoby, 1561)

The clergy of the Anglican Church and lay puritans were equally critical of Englishwomen who adopted the cosmetic arts of Italian women. There is a theory that the Reformation was indirectly to blame for these frivolous innovations. The Dissolution of the Nunneries had increased the number of laywomen in the country and, without an example of religious virtue to emulate, more women were open to the influence of the new ideas in fashion. This theory, although ingenious, seems unlikely in view of the fact that a staunchly Catholic country such as Italy was the prime originator of cosmetic fashions at this period.

In spite of such criticisms as Ben Jonson's:

> Still to be neat, still to be drest,
> As you were going to a feast,
> Still to be powder'd, still perfum'd
> Lady, it is to be presumed,
> though arts hid causes are not found,
> All is not sweet, all is not sound.
> 					(*The Silent Woman*)

Englishwomen, under Elizabeth's leadership, adopted every new cosmetic fashion from the Continent. The fashionable face was achieved by a whole series of preparations. Bearing in mind that the queen's pale complexion was the inspiration for contemporary beauty, it is not surprising that white powder was the foundation on which the rest of the cosmetic treatment was applied. Unfortunately, one of the most successful means of creating a white powder was by using ceruse, or white lead, which was extremely dangerous for the complexion and, if used constantly, had a harmful toxic effect on the individual. This substance formed the basis for cosmetics for several centuries with drastic results, which will be discussed at length in a later chapter. White powder was also made from ground alabaster or starch with perfume added as an ingredient. After the face was powdered, rouge was applied to the cheeks; at this period red ochre was the most popular colourant. Rouge was also made from a white lead base with a colouring dye included in the compound. In either form contemporary rouge had none of the subtlety of its modern equivalent. The lips were painted with a 'pencil' made from ground alabaster or plaster of Paris which was powdered down and mixed into a paste with a colouring ingredient. The mixture was rolled into a crayon shape, then allowed to dry and solidify in the sun.

White powder, rouge and lip colouring formed the basic cosmetic equipment of the fashionable Elizabethan lady. After applying this make-up, she preserved her 'face' by covering her skin with a thin glaze of egg-white and, should she venture out of doors, her artificial complexion was further protected by a mask. The wearing of masks during the Elizabethan period had a dual purpose, first to preserve the face in its original cosmetic perfection and, secondly, to provide protection against the sun which was the chief enemy of a fashionable white complexion. The mask was cut in an oval shape with holes for the eyes, and kept in position by a button held in the teeth.

Elizabethan women were constantly seeking new methods of

preserving or creating a white complexion. Many ingenious recipes were invented by contemporary housewives and by such men as Sir Hugh Platt, whose *Delightes for Ladies*, one of the first household recipe books, appeared in 1602. This included numerous recipes for cosmetics:

To Make a Blanch For any Ladies Face

Of white Tartar take two drams, Camphire one dram, Coperas half a dram, the whites of four Eggs, juice of two lemmons, oyl of Tartar four ounces, Plantan water as much, white Mercury a pennyworth, bitter Almonds two ounces, al must be powdred and mixed with the oyl and water and then boyled upon a gentle fire and strain it, and so keep it: the party must rub her face with a Scarlet cloath and then over night wash her with it, and in the morning wash it off with Bran and white wine.

Another tackles the problem of a freckled skin:

To take away Spots and Freckles from the Face and Hands

The sap that issueth out of a Birch tree in great abundance, being opened in March and Aprill, with a receiver of Glass set under the boring thereof to receive the same doth perfume the same most excellently and maketh the skin very cleer.

A further recipe offers an expedient solution:

To Make the Face White and Fair

Wash they face with Rosemary boyled in white wine, and thou shalt be fair.

White hands were also considered essential to perfect beauty. This was undoubtedly due to the influence of Elizabeth who was justly proud of her delicate, long-fingered white hands, always featured so prominently in her portraits. Hands, as a result, were frequently described in the romantic love poetry of the period.

Full gently now she takes him by the hand,
A lily prison'ed in a gaol of snow,
Or ivory in an alabaster band;
So white a friend engirts so white a foe
(Shakespeare. 'Venus and Adonis')

The high standard of perfection demanded by fashion
depended on a variety of preparations. Ointments and lotions
were concocted from ingredients such as ass's milk, hog lard,
honey and beeswax, with added embellishments of cherries,
rose petals and herbs. Elizabethan ointments and lotions seem
to have contained relatively harmless ingredients. Hog lard,
honey and beeswax may not have improved the condition of
contemporary skins but, unlike ceruse-based cosmetics, they
were not dangerous. Turpentine and rosin were used to cure
blemished complexions. In the latter part of the sixteenth
century, bear's grease formed a basis for some cosmetics. This
was a much safer ingredient than white lead, but proved too
expensive for general use. Olive oil was employed as a basis for
ointments and other cosmetic potions but, although quantities
of oil were imported from Spain and Italy, it never achieved a
lasting popularity. Possibly an oil-based skin lotion attracted
the sun's rays and caused the skin to lose its fashionable
whiteness.

As trade expanded, ingredients for cosmetics and perfumes
came from farther afield and by the middle of the sixteenth
century cargoes of cosmetic materials were imported from all
over the Continent and the Levant. Cochineal and saffron
flowers, henna, Arabian gum and exotic dyes and spices poured
into the country from Marseilles, Italy, Baghdad and Cyprus.
Cosmetic materials were of such interest to Elizabethan England
that an officer on Sir Walter Ralegh's voyage of discovery to
Guiana describes to an 'especiall' friend in London 'Divers
Berryes which dye a most perfect Crimson and Carnation; and
for painting, not all France, Italy nor the East Indies yeeld any

such, for the more the skinne is washed the fairer the colour appeareth'.

Soap was also imported, mainly from Spain and Italy. Castile soap was considered the finest, with Venetian an excellent alternative. English manufactured soap was not fashionable although there were home recipes for making what was frequently described as a 'washing ball':

> Take three ounces of Orace, half an ounce of Cypress, two ounces of Rose leaves, two ounces of Lavender flowers: beat all these together in a Morter, fercing them thorow a fine fearce, then scrape some Castil sope, and dissolve it with some Rose-water and then incorporate all your powders therewith, by labouring them well in a Morter.
>
> (*Delightes for Ladies*)

Although soap was popular at this period, the standards of hygiene were low. Baths were seldom taken except for the medicinal treatment of rheumatism and gout, and as a method of warming cold feet in the winter. 'Cold and naturall bathes are greatly expedient for men subject to rheumes, dropsies and goutes'. (William Vaughn, *Artificial Directions For Health*.) This lack of bathing greatly increased the importance of perfume but, as contemporary scents were composed of fugitive ingredients, repeated applications must have been needed to ensure any degree of freshness.

Elizabeth proved no exception to the general rule concerning baths and, according to contemporary sources, resorted to this drastic means of cleanliness once a month. She probably used one of the many contemporary perfumes and, although historians write that she preferred a light scent, it is possible that a heavier scent with lasting qualities was not available at this period. She made liberal use of rose water which was imported for her from Antwerp, but her own special scent was a delicate mixture of herbs with a predominance of marjoram.

79

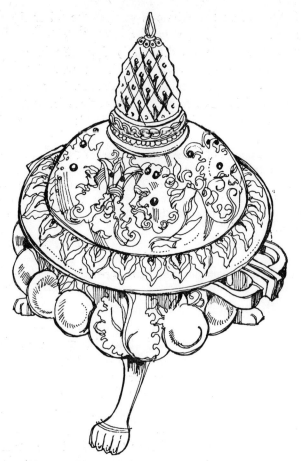

Fig 12 Perfume burner in embossed copper, Italian,
sixteenth century

Scented water was used for washing the face and hands, and
William Vaughn suggests that to 'Wash your face, eyes, eares
and handes with fountaine water' was an agreeable method of
cleansing and beautifying the skin. Etiquette demanded that
hands should be washed before meals as at this period it was

80

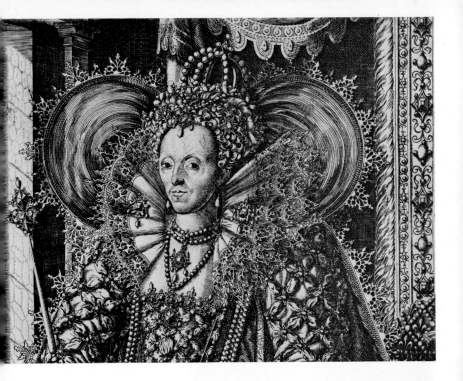

16 (*above*) Queen Elizabeth I. Detail of an engraving, by William Rogers, which illustrates a bizarre cosmetic fashion. The painting of artificial veins on the forehead was probably adopted by Elizabeth in middle age to simulate a youthfully translucent complexion.

17 (*right*) Elizabethan gentleman. A portrait miniature by Nicholas Hilyarde. A perfect representation of the Elizabethan courtier, whose curled locks, well-groomed mustache and whimsically lovesick pose are more reminiscent of an Italian gentleman and indicate the influence Italy had on contemporary looks in England.

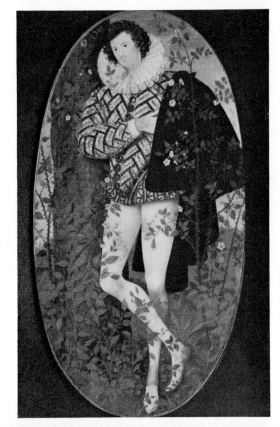

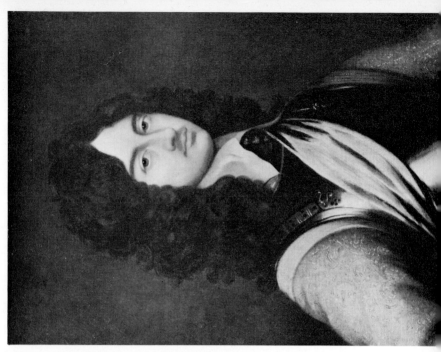

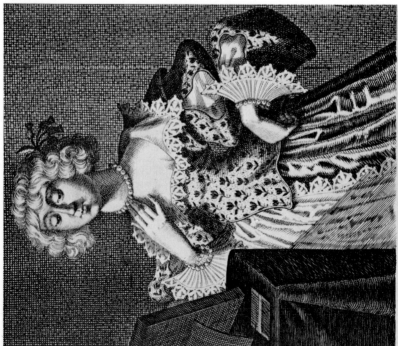

18 (*left*) A lady at her looking glass.

19 (*right*) Charles II as a young man. Portrait by an unknown artist. The elaborately curled shoulder-length hair may well have been a periwig, which was certainly styled in this fashion.

still common to have a dish of food from which everyone helped themselves. 'Before meals it is right to wash your hands openly, even though you have no need to do so, in order that those who dip their fingers in the same dish as yourself may know for certain that you have cleaned them'. (Della Casa. *Galateo*. Mid-sixteenth century.)

Clothes were liberally perfumed after laundering.

A Special Sweet Water to Perfume Clothes in the Folding, being washed

Take a quart of Damask rosewater, and put it into a Glass, put into it a handful of Lavender flowers, two ounces of Orris, a dram of musk, the weight of four-pence of Amber-greece, as much of Civet, four drops of oyl of Cloves; stop this close, and set it in the sun a fortnight; put one spoonful of this water into a Glass, and so sprinkle your clothes therewith in your folding.

(*Delightes for Ladies*)

Gloves, which were an important fashion accessory, were also scented and so were handkerchiefs.

A noticeable aspect of the appearance and an important item of personal hygiene were the teeth. Their condition, due to an unbalanced diet and unhealthy living standards, was deplorable. 'If she have black and rugged Teeth, let her offer the less a laughter, especially if she laugh wide and open'. (Ben Jonson. *The Silent Woman*.)

Teeth were cleaned by rubbing them with a linen cloth, after which the mouth was rinsed out with a mouth wash. William Vaughn, writing in 1600, gives an ingenious, if ineffective, routine for dental care:

Pick and rub your teeth and because I would not have you bestow much cost in making dentifrices, I will advertise you by foure rules of importance how to keep your teeth white and uncorrupt, and also have a sweet breath. First wash well your mouth when you have eaten your meate, secondly sleepe with your mouth somewhat open. Thirdly spit out in the morning . . . then take a linnen cloth and rub your teeth well within and without to take away the fumositie of the meate and the yellownesse of the teeth.

The mouth wash consisted of:

½ a glass of vinegar and as much of the water of the masticke tree, of rosemarie, mirrhe, masticke, bole, Arkmoniake, Dragon's herbe, roche allome of each of them an ounce, and of fountain water three glassfulles; mingle all well together, and let it boile with a final fire, adding to it halfe a pound of honie, and taking away the scum of it, then put in a little bengwine, and when it hath sodden a quarter of an houre, take it from the fire, and keepe it in a cleane bottle and wash your teeth therewithall.

Sir Hugh Platt describes a 'sweet and delicate dentifrice, or rubbers for the Teeth':

Dissolve in four ounces of warm water three or four drams of Gumdragagant, and in one night this will become a little substance like a gelly; mingle the same with the powder of Alabaster finely ground and fearsed, then make up this substance into little round rouls, of the bigness of a child's arrow.

Mouth washes, dentrifrices and sucking jewels were employed to keep the mouth fresh, but the most popular and expedient form of dental care was the toothpick. Elizabethan toothpicks were made of gold, silver, ivory or hartshorn. A New Year's gift to Elizabeth included a selection of gold toothpicks and linen rubbing cloths edged in black and silver. A toothpick was frequently carried on the person, but as Della Casa writes in the *Galateo*:

Anyone who carries a toothpick hung on a cord around his neck is certainly at fault, for besides the fact that it is a strange object to see drawn from beneath a gentleman's waistcoat and reminds us of those cheapjack dentists who can be seen in the market-place, it also shows that the wearer is well-equipped and provided with the wherewithall of a glutton.

Hair cleanliness was another problem. Headdresses diminished in importance towards the end of the sixteenth century and were replaced by elaborately curled hairstyles built up over padding and wire frames. The focus on hair meant that it had to be kept in good condition. The most popular method of cleaning hair was by the use of 'lye', a compound of wood ash and water. 'You shall find it wonderful expedient, if you bath your head foure times in the yeere and with hot lie made from ashes.' (William Vaughn. *Artificial Directions for Health.*)

It was essential that hair should be the right fashionable colour. Elizabeth's own naturally red hair set the pattern for the rest of female society, but golden hair was also popular due to the influence of the Italian court. Dyes were used to colour hair 'a fair yellow or golden colour'; and 'the Dog berry is an excellent berry to make a golden liquor withal for this purpose'. (*Delightes for Ladies.*) Another recipe suggests that after washing the hair 'by a good fire in warm Allom water

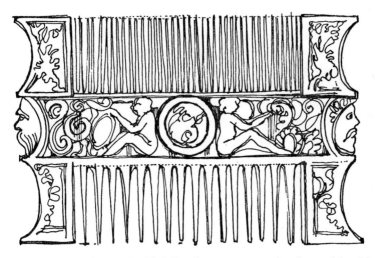

Fig 13 Ivory comb carved with foliated ornament, putti and roundels with male and female busts, German, *c* 1520

83

with a sponge, you may moisten the same in a decoction of Tumerick, Rubarb or the bark of the Barberry tree, and so it will receive a most fair and beautiful colour'. A dye for red hair employs the use of 'the last water that is drawn from Honey, being of a deep red colour, performeth the same excellently but the same hath a strong smell'. (*Delightes for Ladies.*)

With middle age, Elizabeth's hair decreased in quantity and lost its youthful fiery glow. Loss of colour could be replaced by dyes, but its poor quality made it difficult to dress into the fashionable curled style. Elizabeth therefore took to wearing wigs and society ladies followed her example. Although red-haired wigs like the queen's were the most popular, blonde wigs were also worn.

> Her hair is auburn, mine a perfect yellow
> If that be all the difference in his love
> I'll get me such a colour'd periwig.
> (Shakespeare. *Two Gentlemen of Verona*)

Many portraits of Elizabethan women with red hair have been mistaken for Elizabeth, but it is probable that a wig camouflaged their own colouring and gave them a startling likeness to the queen.

Elizabeth had a comprehensive selection of wigs and in 1602 it is recorded that she purchased six heads of hair, twelve yards of hair curl and a hundred other devices made of hair. She also possessed a massive wardrobe of dresses and every form of cosmetic preparation common to the age. Many of her cosmetics were prepared by herself and she favoured a strange assortment of ingredients. She was reputed to have used the fat of a puppy dog mixed with apples to make a hair pomade, a compound of posset curd to free her forehead from wrinkles, and an elaborate skin lotion included egg-white, powdered egg shells, alum, borax and white poppy seeds.

Her face make-up of white powder, rouge and lip dye glazed with egg white had set the fashion for other Elizabethan women. She also plucked her eyebrows and forehead to reveal a greater expanse of white skin, a medieval habit that persisted throughout the Tudor and Elizabethan periods. To draw attention to her high plucked forehead and to simulate the translucency of a perfect white skin, Elizabeth even painted artificial veins on her brow (*Plate 16*). This quaint cosmetic device was most probably used to replace, in middle age, the natural beauty of a youthful complexion. Cosmetics and scents were imported for Elizabeth from all over the Continent and, as she grew older, she tried many lotions and elixirs that purported to preserve or recreate youth. A Dutch physician became extremely unpopular with Elizabeth when his elixir of youth had no effect and from then on she reposed her confidence in the eccentric contemporary alchemist Dr John Dee.

Elizabeth's vanity influenced the whole environment of court life. Personal appearance was of such prime importance that it resulted in an increased sale of mirrors. At the beginning of the sixteenth century mirrors were an unusual luxury, but at the end of Elizabeth's reign they had become a universal necessity. They were manufactured in the Netherlands and in Venice and, as the century progressed, became more elaborate in design. Pocket mirrors made of polished steel or glass also became fashionable. These items of personal conceit were vital equipment to the Elizabethan courtier.

This was undoubtedly the age of the courtier. The chivalrous knight of the Middle Ages, with his formal ritual of courtly love, was replaced by a lighter-hearted individual who owed more to wit than convention. His gallantry towards women still followed a prescribed pattern and it is interesting that two Italian works of social etiquette were translated into English at this period. Count Baldassare Castiglione's *Book of the Courtier* was translated by Sir Thomas Hoby in 1561 and the first English version of Della Casa's *Galateo* was dedicated to that most famous of courtiers, Robert Dudley, Earl of Leicester.

Englishmen owed much to an Italian influence in social behaviour and dress:

> Report of fashions in proud Italy
> Whose manners still our tardy apish nation
> Limps after in base imitation
> (Shakespeare. *Richard II*)

and, although a puritanically English element of society ridiculed the extreme fashions in Italian dress and etiquette, the majority of sophisticated Englishmen followed the example set by Italian courtiers.

Nicholas Hillyarde painted a perfect picture of the young courtier in a delightful miniature of this period (*Plate 17*). He captured the whole spirit of the romantic Elizabethan age in the whimsically lovesick pose of his subject:

> His browny locks did hang in crooked curls
> And every light occasion of the wind
> Upon his lips their silken parcels hurls
> (Shakespeare. 'A Lover's Complaint')

The English courtier wore his hair moderately long and curled; while his moustache and pointed beard were groomed into a perfect shape and kept in place with the aid of gum. He used hair pomades and scent to make himself agreeable to ladies and wore perfumed gloves to protect his white hands from the elements. Real dandies carried fans and exquisite lace handkerchiefs; they also wore make-up, a habit which Shakespeare found disgusting and unmanly. Fops who persisted in any excessive use of artifice to improve their appearance were severely criticised by the rest of society. 'A man ought not to embellish himself like a woman . . . I sometimes

86

see men whose hair and beards are curled with hot tongs and whose face, necks and hands have been smoothed and titivated more than any young wench'. (*Galateo.*) Cosmetics were not generally used by truly masculine courtiers, but the application of too much perfume came in for criticism. 'There should be no excessive smell about the body, either pleasant or otherwise, in order that a gentleman should not have the odour of a workman nor a man carry with him the scent of a woman or a whore'. (*Galateo.*)

It appears that hair-dyeing for men was not unknown at this period and may have been an acceptable form of cosmetic artifice, since recipes for male hair colourants appear amongst conventional household recipes:

How to colour the head or beard into a Chestnut Colour in half an
hour

Take one part of Lead calcined with Sulphur, and one part of quick lime; temper them somewhat thin with water; lay it upon the hair, chafing it well in, and let it dry one quarter of an hour, or thereabout; then wash the same off with fair water divers times; and lastly with sope and water, and it will be a very natural hair colour: the longer it lieth upon the hair, the browner it groweth.

(*Delightes for Ladies*)

The Elizabethan man was certainly more inclined towards 'feminine' ways than his early Tudor forebear and this was probably due to the atmosphere of court life which was orientated to the whims and desires of a woman. Paradoxically, one feels that Elizabeth's feminine nature was responsible for the excessive masculinity of Elizabethan men, who combined sophistication and a delightful protective courtesy towards women with a virile sense of enterprise. Sir Philip Sidney could be described as the ideal example of an Elizabethan gentleman, combining the art of writing exquisite love poems with a spirit of adventure and masculine talent for soldiery.

The dual nature of Elizabethan men derived from the liberated climate of the Tudor and Elizabethan age. The intellect, freed from the mentally confined world of the Middle Ages, inspired a spirit of adventure, sensitivity of imagination and love of beauty. Above all it seems that the Elizabethans had a great appreciation for the trivial as well as the serious aspects of life. They understood that profound talent could be combined with an enjoyment of the frivolous, which explains why, in a climate of intellectual precocity, extravagant fashions flourished and personal beauty was enhanced by the artful embellishments of powder and paint.

CHAPTER SIX

The Seventeenth Century

They will have it, that Painting the Face is against the Seventh Commandment, forbidding all Adultery, for they suppose Painting the Face to be no less than a degree beyond Fornication. (Puritan attitude)

Another reason, that Painting the Face is commendable if not necessary in Woman, is, that the Sex was created in a perfect State of Beauty, and wou'd have continued so in Paradise; So that it is no ignoble Ambition if the Sex aim to evade that Defect which the Fall brought on their Form. (Anglican attitude)

(Attributed to Jeremy Taylor. *Several Letters between Two Ladies wherein the Lawfulness and Unlawfulness of Artificial Beauty In Point of Conscience are Nicely Debated*)

The reign of the first Stuart, James I, was strongly influenced by the Elizabethan way of life, but the spirit of the old court was corrupted into a caricature of its former self. While effecting all the airs and graces of the dandy, the courtier of the Jacobean period lacked the qualities of the true Elizabethan courtier. The underlying virility of the Elizabethan man was replaced by the feminine manner of a *mignon* and undoubtedly the king's homosexual reputation encouraged effeminacy at court.

It is certain that James I's favourites used more make-up than the most flamboyant of Elizabethan fops, and he was reputed to have

> kept a brace of painted creatures to be at his hand
> And be drunk in a new tavern till he be not able to stand.
>   (contemporary popular ballad)

89

The Jacobean dandy practised innumerable affectations with the aid of scent bottles, fans and perfumed gloves, while a single lock of his hair was allowed to remain at shoulder length where it was tied with a silk ribbon. This was the only fashion innovation introduced by James I and was rather preciously described as a 'love lock'.

When Charles I came to the throne in 1625, the court, influenced by the French taste of his queen, Henrietta Maria, adopted Continental fashions in dress and cosmetics. Contemporary hairstyles showed a preference for a softer silhouette, and both sexes wore their hair long and curled to the shoulders, although male courtiers still tied one frond of hair into the Jacobean 'lovelock'.

Fashions had changed drastically from the Elizabethan period, but many cosmetics remained similar to those of the previous century. Ceruse powder, lip dyes and rouge, which still constituted the basic facial cosmetics, were applied with unprecedented generosity, culminating in an extreme of artifice during the Restoration period. Cosmetics had played an important part in the liberated world of Elizabethan England, but in the seventeenth century, in spite of the Puritan influence, cosmetic artifice was more generally accepted due to the Stuarts' close contact with the French court. New fashions in dress and cosmetics frequently originated in Paris society and were quickly adopted by the fashion-conscious in England. This French influence continued to be effective throughout the century, in spite of the restrictions imposed by a civil war and a Puritan dictatorship.

The close link with France and the Continent encouraged increased trade in cosmetic ingredients. Barrel loads of orange flower water, apricot face cream and exotic Parisian powders and perfumes were imported from France. The Netherlands supplied Hungary water, jessemy oil, perfumes and wash balls. Dutch trade with the East Indies produced cargoes of new cosmetic ingredients and the Levant Company imported even more exotic ingredients from Turkey and the Middle East. Trade with India supplied sandalwood, turmeric and musk, and Crete produced quantities of pumice stones. Italy contributed perfumes, essences, oils, toilet water and cochineal, and other cosmetic ingredients and preparations came from Spain and Portugal.

Soap was still imported in great quantities from Castile and Venice, but London manufacturers also produced three varieties: speckled soap, which was worth £6 a ton in 1635; white soap, worth £4 a ton, and grey soap used in cloth manufacture. In 1638 the soapers were incorporated as a City company although they possessed neither hall nor livery. William Noy, a lawyer, introduced his famous 'Project of Soap' at this time. This was designed to produce a revenue from this article by granting a monopoly to the Corporation of Soap Boilers, who had to pay a duty of £8 per ton on all soap manufactured, plus a substantial sum for their right of patent. The industry had become sufficiently productive for Charles I to be able to sell these monopoly rights, but it made him unpopular with rival soap manufacturers, who were well represented in Parliament, and this added to the friction between the Puritan element in Parliament and the king. Although English soap was considered inferior in quality to the Castilian or Venetian equivalent, London manufacturers continued to sell large quantities and by the end of the century there were over sixty soap factories in England.

The manufacture of mirrors became a thriving light industry in seventeenth-century England and manufacturers united to prevent them being imported from the Continent (*Plate 18*). Looking glasses had become increasingly popular since Elizabeth's reign and were brought in from the Netherlands, Venice and Paris, which was also the chief source of the pocket mirror, an essential toilet accessory. Seventeenth-century looking glasses were much more elaborately designed than those of the Elizabethan period and were manufactured with exquisitely moulded frames. They were frequently given as gifts and Ralph Verney of Claydon bought Lady Sussex a mirror from Venice which cost £40.

The increased import of cosmetic materials, soap and mirrors from the Continent, coupled with their extensive manufacture in England, illustrates the importance of personal vanity in the seventeenth century. Men and women spent large sums of money on cosmetic preparations and devoted unlimited time and attention to their *toilette*. Women's faces were liberally powdered with white lead powder, their lips were dyed red and their cheeks amply rouged. In addition, their cheeks were frequently 'patched' with small spots of velvet, leather or even paper. This extraordinary fashion became particularly important in the Restoration period and the eighteenth century. The hair of both sexes was crimped and curled, and often it was powdered, although hair powder was not in general use until a later date. Perfume was used in liberal quantities and every item of clothing was heavily scented.

Excessive cosmetic artificiality and an exaggerated attention to personal vanity have become historically synonymous with the dashing cavalier and his lady. It is, however, as wrong to assume that all royalist sympathisers approved of artificial beauty as it is to suppose that all contemporary puritans abandoned every form of fashionable artifice. Certainly the true Presbyterian puritan left his hair uncurled and in many cases it was cropped short, hence the followers of Oliver Cromwell were aptly known as 'Crop Ears' or 'Roundheads'. Women frequently concealed their hair under a bonnet and puritan hat, and left their faces unpainted.

Jeremy Taylor, a distinguished prelate and protégé of Archbishop Laud, was reputed to have written an amusing dialogue between an Anglican lady and a Puritan lady in which they discuss artificial beauty. Although it is in Taylor's style, there is a theory that his wife may have written the dialogue as a practical joke. It was entitled *Several Letters between Two Ladies wherein the Lawfulness and Unlawfulness of Artificial Beauty in Point of Conscience Are Nicely Debated. Published for the satisfaction of the Fair Sex.* It illustrated to perfection the opposing viewpoints of royalist and puritan. The puritan lady opens the discussion: 'Persons of Quality, who not content with Nature's stock of Beauty, do (not by a fine, but filthy art) add something to the advantage, as they think, of their Complexions; but, I fear, to the deforming of their Souls'. The 'royalist' lady argues that any Puritan would use medicine to combat disease and 'Only in the point of Colour or Tinctures, added in the least kind or degree, they are not more scrupulous than censorious; as if every one that used these had forsaken Christ's banner, and now fought under the Devil's colours'.

> *Puritan lady:* 'Truly, Madam, I absolutely think (without mincing or distinction) all Colour or Complexion added to our Skins or faces, beyond what is purely natural, to be a sin, as being flatly against the Word of God . . . Jezebel, though a Queen, was yet not tolerated or excused, but foully branded and heavily punished for painting her eyes or face.'
>
> *Royalist lady:* 'Among which this of her painting is indeed set down chiefly, to shew, that no advantage of outward Beauty, *natural* or artificial (though set off with the Curiosity and Majesty of a Queen) are sufficient to make any Person the object of either Love or Pity.'
>
> *Puritan lady:* 'But Painting the face, good Madam, is mentioned in two other places of Scripture, as the practice of Lewd and Wicked Women.'

The answer which the 'royalist' lady gives at this point in the conversation criticises the double standards of many puritans who, although against the use of cosmetics, were content to comfort themselves with other vanities and luxuries:

93

If your Ladiship thinks the sharp stile of that place strikes so severely against all Painting and Complexioning as a Sin, why may you not also by the same severity destroy and disallow all other things there expressed in the same Tone and Tenour? As dressing and decking yourself with any costly and comely ornaments, all sweet perfumes, all sitting on rich and stately beds, with tables before them . . . I will not captiously reply upon your Ladiship, by putting you to plead for your own and your children's wearing of well-set, curled, gummed, braided and powdered hair . . . nor will I retort upon your gold jewels, ear-rings and costly apparel . . . are more expressly against the Letter of those Scriptures, than anything you have yet urged against Tincture or Complexioning.

But the puritan lady, with the single-mindedness of a true bigot, can only repeat the same accusation against the use of cosmetics: 'But, good Madam, laying side the Flourishes of Wit and Colours of Speech, (whereof I am not prone to be guilty) in Plain English, Ought not a Christian to rest humbly content and satisfied with the Will of God, submitting thereto without any such contending in patching and painting ways'.

The viewpoint of the puritan lady in this dialogue would have been strongly upheld by Oliver Cromwell and in the year after Charles I's execution, a bill was introduced to Parliament against 'the Vice of Painting and wearing black Patches and immodest Dresses of Women'. Although this bill never became an act, from this date onwards, during the exile of the Stuart court, the Puritans labelled as prostitutes all women who used cosmetics. Parliament also levied a heavy tax on soap, which continued until the Restoration of Charles II in 1660.

During this period of oppressive Parliament rule, many ardent royalists followed the young future king to exile in France. The Verneys of Claydon were one such family and it is probably due to these exiles that so many new cosmetic ideas were introduced into England after the Restoration. One French fashion which fascinated Sir Ralph Verney was the periwig which provided men with an excellent substitute for a natural curled coiffure. 'Let it be well curled in great rings and not frizzled and see that he makes it handsomely and fashionably, and with two locks, and let them be tyed with black ribbon'. (Verney Memoirs.) This edifice of hair would have cost Sir Ralph twelve livres at this time. Natural hair was cropped short under the wig to ensure a close fit. The French prided themselves on the invention of such a hygienic fashion, as long hair was difficult to keep clean due to the inefficiency of soap. Royalist families in exile, though hampered by low finances, endeavoured to keep up with French fashions and Sir Ralph Verney was determined that his wife should have a good supply of 'pomatums . . . pinns, oris powder and such matters' sent from London. The exiles also supplied their friends in England with French cosmetic preparations. Sir John Cooke, writing to an English friend, asks him to give a present of French hair powder to a lady: ' a small phiole of white Cyprus powder, which I beseech you present to my Lady as an example of the best Montpelier affords, for I saw it made myself. It must be mixed with other powder, else it will bring the headache. There is powder cheaper, but not so proper for the hair'. (Verney Memoirs); and an English friend writing to Sir Ralph Verney asks him to find out about the new French fashion of 'little brushes for making cleane of the teeth, most covered with gold and sylver Twiste together with some petits Bouettes [boxes] to put them in.' (Verney Memoirs.)

In the year 1660, the exiled Stuart court returned to England and Charles II was crowned in Westminster Abbey. Royalist supporters made every effort to ensure that the coronation was a suitably lavish affair and families participating in the procession celebrated the occasion by spending exorbitant sums of money on clothing for themselves and their retinues. The Earl of Bedford spent £1,000 on dress for his retinue and this did not include clothing for his immediate family. This unprecedented display of extravagance set the tone for the rest of the century and society reacted against the restrictive period of puritanism by indulging in extremes of fashion in dress and cosmetic artifice. Vanity was no longer a vice but a desirable virtue.

The contemporary ideal of beauty was perfectly represented in the portraits by Peter Lely. The women, in flowing silk dresses enhanced with delicate lace and with their hair softly curled, have a look of subtle sensuality. Their complexions are rose-tinted and their features generously moulded, with soft red lips and dark luminous eyes more reminiscent of French than of English beauty.

The king collaborated with his subjects in their efforts to dispel the blight of puritanism from England and introduced many exotic fashions inspired by ideas gleaned from the French court (*Plate 19*). The periwig became an essential accessory and, for the first time in history, wigs were worn as an item of fashion in their own right rather than as a means of disguising loss of hair. They cost vast sums of money and, in 1672, the Earl of Bedford paid his wigmaker £54 10s for four periwigs which individually cost £20, £18, £10 and £6. Contemporary drama alluded to the cost of wigs. 'Perriwigs so dear, that the Devil take me, I am reduc'd to that extremity in my cash, I have been forc'd to rentrench in that one Article of Sweet Pawder, till I have braught it dawn to Five Guineas a Month . . . Now judge, Tam, whether I can spare you Five Hundred Pounds.' (Sir John Vanbrugh. *The Relapse*.) Quantities of women's hair were imported to supplement local supplies used in the manufacture of wigs, but the periwig nearly went out of fashion during the Great Plague of London in 1665 when 'nobody will dare to buy any haire for fear of the infection, that it had been cut off the heads of people dead of the plague'. (Samuel Pepys. *Diary*.) However, even the risk of deadly disease did not dissuade society from relying on their false hair once the initial fear had been surmounted by vanity.

96

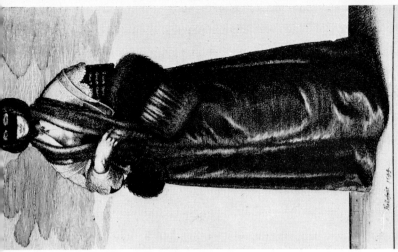

The Winter habit
of ane English Gentlewoman.

of her face with its red lips and heavy-lidded eyes typifies the kind of beauty favoured during the Restoration period. She painted her face liberally for her theatrical performances.

21 (*right*) 'The Winter Habit of an English Gentlewoman'. Engraving by Hollar (1607–77). Masks were worn to protect the complexion from sunburn. Men also wore them; the expression 'bare-faced' dates from this time when few members of society ventured into the London streets with their faces uncovered.

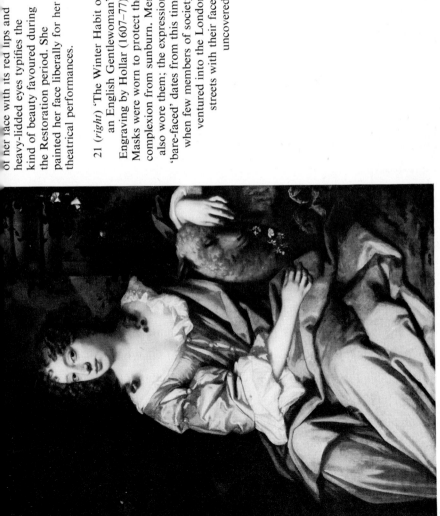

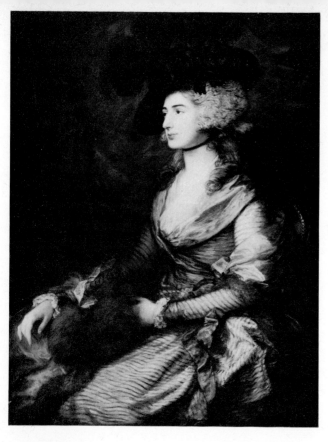

22 (*left*) Mrs Siddons. Portrait by Thomas Gainsborough whose paintings conveyed the impression that eighteenth-century women possessed naturally beautiful 'English rose' complexions, an idea which was contradicted by the contemporary caricaturist.

23 (*below*) 'Dressing for a Birthday'. Caricature by Thomas Rowlandson. Contemporary woman seen through the eyes of a satirical artist. Note the 'patched' cheeks; patches hid disfiguring marks left by smallpox

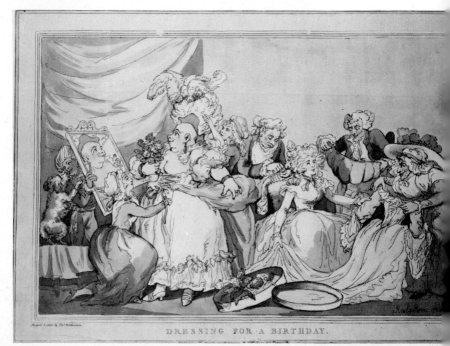

DRESSING FOR A BIRTHDAY.

Women rarely wore full wigs at this period, but their natural hair was supplemented with false pieces and curled into the semblance of an artificial concoction. Foreheads were plucked and decorated with spirals of hair described as *Favorites*. Curls were extremely popular and appeared in every shape and form

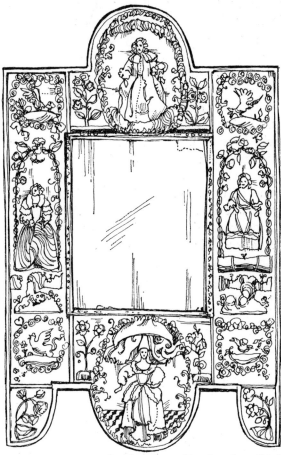

Fig 14 Nell Gwyn's looking glass of beadwork, padded to represent figures, with silver braid edging, English, mid-seventeenth century

as a decorative device. *The Fop's Dictionary* of 1700 describes, amongst other fashionable affectations, '*Les Meurtrières*—Murderers; a certain knot in the Hair, which ties and unites the Curls' and '*Le Creve-Coeur*—Heartbreakers, the two small curl'd Locks at the Nape of the Neck'.

The extravagant quality of contemporary hairstyles was echoed in the artificial ornamentation of the face. Cosmetics were used to an unprecedented degree and, to modern eyes, the late-seventeenth-century face would have appeared theatrically over-painted. It is possible that theatrical make-up did influence many women in their use of cosmetics. Judging by Pepys's *Diary*, society spent a great deal of time at the theatre where, for the first time in English dramatic history, actresses instead of young actors could be seen playing female roles. At a time when novelty was thought a virtue, actresses were a delightful innovation and Charles II set an example to the rest of society by courting one of the most popular comediennes of her day, Nell Gwyn (*Plate 20*). Her success with the king resulted in actresses being accepted as 'fringe' members of society and well-born ladies may well have copied from them the exaggerations of stage make-up in their own daily use of cosmetics. It is certain that actresses were heavily painted for their theatrical performances. Pepys writes of Nell Gwyn and Mrs Knipp, another popular actress, 'But, Lord! to see how they were both painted would make a man mad, and did make me loathe them'.

The contemporary face was blanched with powder and the cheeks were dyed with 'Spanish leather' rouge from Seville. 'Spanish leather' was a piece of scarlet leather (the alternative was 'Spanish paper'), which coloured the skin on application. Blemishes, such as spots or pock marks, were hidden by an exotic array of 'patches' shaped like stars or crescent moons. It is interesting that these were cut out in such obviously oriental symbols, in view of the Eastern influence in male costume currently described as 'The Persian Mode' (John

Evelyn). The artificial complexion was still protected out of doors by a mask; this contemporary equivalent of the Elizabethan fashion was described as a 'Loo Mask' and covered only half the face. The fact that this half-mask offered less protection was perhaps of secondary importance at a time when coquetry in women was desirable and the 'Loo Mask', which offered a half-veiled glimpse of identity, created endless possibilities for seductive flirtation (*Plate 21*). Men also wore masks and the expression 'bare-faced' originates from this period when few members of society ventured into the London streets with their faces uncovered. Ornate fans were used for the same purpose as masks.

An unblemished skin was a rarity at this period, but every attempt was made to acquire and preserve a pure, pale complexion. Charles II's queen, Catherine of Braganza, was never considered very attractive by the English because her skin colouring was dark.

> The Queen arrived with a train of Portuguese ladies in their monstrous fardingales or guard-infantes their complexions olivarder [olive-coloured] and sufficiently unagreeable. Her Majesty in the same habit, her fore-top long and turned aside very strangely. She was yet of the handsomest countenance of all the rest, and, though low of stature, prettily shaped, languishing and excellent eyes, her teeth wronging her mouth by sticking a little too far out; for the rest, lovely enough. (John Evelyn. *Diary*)

John Evelyn's assessment of Catherine's looks was far more charitable than that of his contemporaries, but even he mentioned her outmoded dress and unfashionably dark skin. The king, however, seemed delighted with his young queen whose childlike vulnerability may have appealed to his masculine sense of gallantry: 'I can only give you an account of what I have seen abed, which in shorte is, her face is not so exact as to be called a beauty, though her eyes are excellent good, and not anything in her face that in the least degree can shoque

99

one'. Unfortunately for the queen, his appreciation of feminine qualities was not restricted to her alone and during his lifetime he formed many liaisons with other women. His mistresses were a considerable drain on the king's purse, as alimonies had to compensate for royal indiscretions and presents were expected as tokens of the king's esteem. Such gifts as apricot paste and other costly ointments were highly prized by the recipients as cosmetics had soared in price after the Restoration.

Expensive cosmetic items were acquired by most members of society, and exotic or exclusive preparations were regarded as a form of 'status symbol'. Home-made lotions and ointments were also in evidence. An interesting correspondence between Lady Sussex and her friends, the Verneys, illustrates the use of home recipes for beauty: 'The fines thing that can be my cosen baron sayeth is poset curd with red rose lefes boyled in the milke and torned with ale' and 'Myrrh water is good to make on lok younge longe; I only wete a fine cloth and wipe my face over at night with it.' (Verney Memoirs.) These two recipes seem very Elizabethan in content; perhaps seventeenth-century men and women believed their forebears had a special talent in this field. There may be, for this reason, a connection between Elizabeth I's pomade, reputedly made from puppy dog fat, and the unsavoury seventeenth-century belief that drinking puppy dog urine was good for the complexion. Puppy dog fat was also used in contemporary recipes:

To Make Pig, or Puppidog Water for the Face

Take a Fat Pig, or a Fat Puppidog, of nine days old, and kill it, order it as to Roast, save the Blood, and fling away nothing but the Guts; then take the Blood, and Pig or the Puppidog, and break the Legs and Head, with all the Liver and the rest of the Inwards, of either of them put all into the still if it will hold it, to that, take two Quarts of old Canary, a pound of unwash'd Butter not salted; a Quart of Snails-shells, and also two Lemmons, only the outside pared away; Still all these together in a Rose Water Still,

100

either at once or twice; Let it drop slowly into a Glass-Bottle, in which there be a lump of Loaf-Sugar, and a little Leaf-gold. (*The Lady's Dressing Room Unlock'd and The Fop's Dictionary*, 1700)

The use of such toxic ingredients in cosmetic preparations and a generally low standard of hygiene resulted in early loss of beauty: 'they cry a Woman's past her prime at twenty, Decay'd at four and twenty, old and unsufferable at thirty' (Sir George Etherege. *The Man of Mode*.) Society women were therefore anxious to find any means of prolonging their youthful looks as

> The deprav'd apetite of this Vicious Age
> Tastes nothing but green Fruit, and loathes it when
> Tis' kindly ripen'd.
>
> (*The Man of Mode*)

This desire to remain beautiful made contemporary women particularly gullible to the promises of a charlatan physician, Dr Alexander Bendo, who elected to cure blemished complexions with his miraculous concoctions. When Bendo set up his business in a goldsmith's house in London, in the guise of an 'Italian doctor', society did not guess the true identity of this enigmatical man of medicine. Bendo was none other than the eccentric young Earl of Rochester who had been banished from court circles for writing a rude lampoon against Charles II. A worse fate than banishment would have awaited the earl had he not been the king's ward, but Rochester's restive nature did not take kindly to enforced exile in the country and a return to society in disguise appealed to his daredevil spirit and sense of humour. It also put him in contact with numerous society ladies. Whilst at court, Rochester had acquired a considerable reputation as a rake; his sexual appetites had extended to all levels of society from aristocratic women to serving wenches, whom he frequently seduced disguised as a court servant. Therefore, in his new guise of 'doctor', his 'patients' trusted him as an honourable medical man. His ability in amateur chemistry made it possible for him to create cosmetic preparations, whose effectiveness was largely an illusion imbued with credibility by 'Bendo's' claims of success on the Continent:

> The knowledge of these secrets, I gathered in my travels abroad (where I have spent my time ever since I was fifteen years old, to this my nine and twentieth year) in France and Italy. Those that have travelled in Italy, will tell you what a miracle art does there assist Nature in the preservation of beauty; how women of forty bear the same countenance with those of fifteen: ages are no way distinguished by faces; whereas here in England, look a horse in the mouth, and a woman in the face, you presently know both their ages to a year. I will, therefore, give you such remedies, that, without destroying your complexion (as most paints and daubings do), shall render them perfectly fair; clearing and preserving them from all spots, freckles, heats, pimples and marks of the small-pox, or any other accidental ones, so that the face be not seamed or scarred.

Like most capricious characters, Rochester tired of his new role after a time and returned to the country. He was eventually pardoned by the king, but only survived to the age of thirty-three when he died of a fever.

Nicholas Culpeper, a contemporary physician and herbalist, employed his more genuine talents to compile a book of herbal medicines and beauty preparations, which were based on the writings of Pliny and Hippocrates. The *Physician and Herbal* listed numerous natural remedies in which even the most commonplace wild plants were used as ingredients. 'The Teasle: The distilled water of the leaves is often used by women to preserve their beauty' and 'The Elm Tree: The water that is found in the bladders of the leaves while it is fresh, is very effectual to cleanse the skin and make it fair'. It is a lasting tribute to the effective quality of Culpeper's preparations that his herbal cosmetics, based on the original recipes, are still popular today.

The importance of cosmetics at this period meant that much time was spent in the boudoir experimenting with new preparations and perfumes. This obsessive preoccupation with personal vanity aroused criticism of an unfashionably puritanical nature in Sir George Savile, first Marquis of Halifax, who wrote a

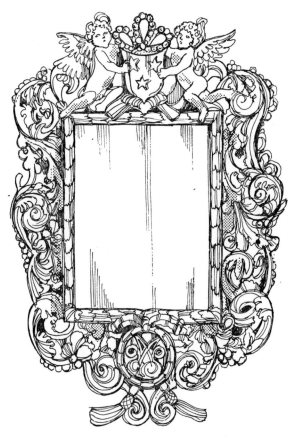

Fig 15 Carved pine-wood wall mirror, stained and partly gilt. At the top, two *amorini* support a shield bearing the arms of the Hildyard family of Winestead Hall, Yorkshire, English, *c* 1670

103

book for his daughter entitled *The Lady's New Year's Gift* in which he condemned the vain woman: 'The Looking glass in the morning dictateth to her all the Motions of the Day, which by how much the more studied, are so much the more mistaken' and 'She doth not like herself as God Almighty made her, but will have some of her own Workmanship; which is so far from making her a better thing than a woman that it turneth her into a worse Creature than a Monkey'. These criticisms may have had an effect on Savile's daughter, but the majority of society women and men continued to spend several hours of the day in the boudoir. While they completed this lengthy *toilette*, they diverted themselves by entertaining society friends; this was the origin of the *levee* or 'toilet gathering' which became an essential part of social life during the eighteenth century. Thus dressing rooms in most society residences assumed the importance of a major reception room and were decorated accordingly, with costly silk hangings and pictures which suited the taste of the individual. The Earl of Bedford had his toilet table covered in pale blue silk with a pin-cushion and comb bags in matching fabric, the whole of which cost forty-five shillings in 1670. Boudoir looking glasses were frequently given as gifts at this time and Catherine of Braganza received from the queen mother, Henrietta Maria, 'the great looking-glass and toilet of beaten and massive gold'. (John Evelyn, *Diary*.) On the toilet tables were beautiful boxes made of precious metals, bottles of French perfumes and numerous pots of cosmetics:

> A new Scene to us next presents,
> The Dressing-Room, and Implements,
> Of Toilet Plate Gilt and Emboss'd,
> And several other things of Cost,
> The Table miroir, one Glue Pot,
> One for Pomatum, and what not,
> Of Washes, Unguents, and Cosmeticks,
> Snuffers, and Snuff-dish, Boxes more,

For Powders, Patches, Waters store,
In Silver Flasks, or bottles, Cups
Cover'd or open to wash chaps.
   (*The Lady's Dressing Room Unlock'd*)

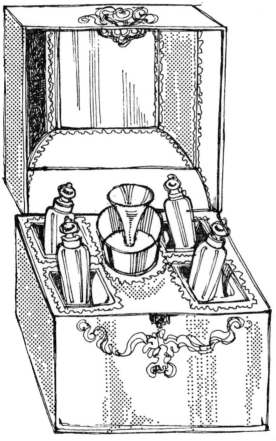

Fig 16 Perfume essence case covered in leather with silver mounts, and fitted with four cut-glass silver-stoppered flasks, a silver measure and a funnel, Dutch, late seventeenth century

The boudoir was heavily perfumed with the scent of aromatic powder, which was liberally sprinkled all over the room and its contents, and perfumed 'sweet bags' made of sarcenet were laid amongst clothes and linen to keep them fresh:

> In Amber'd Skins or quilted chest
> Richly perfume'd, She Lays, and rare
> Powders for Garments, Some for Hair
> Of Cyprus and of Corduba,
> And the Rich Polvil of Goa,
> Nor here omit the Bob of Gold
> Which a Pomander Ball does hold
> . . .
> A large rich cloth of Gold toilet
> Does cover, and to put Rags
> Two high embroider'd Sweet Bags.
> (*The Lady's Dressing Room Unlock'd*)

A great variety of perfumes and essences were available at this period; and men and women acquired a selection of scents to suit their personal taste. The Earl of Bedford used both orange flower water and Queen of Hungary water as 'after shave' lotions, and other scents were:

> Twelve dozen Martial, whole and half,
> Of Jonquil, Tuberose (don't laugh)
> Frangipan, Orange, Violett,
> Narcissus, Jassemin, Ambrett

and

> D'ange, Orange, Mill-Fleur, Myrtle
> Whole Quarts the chamber to bespertle.
> (*The Lady's Dressing Room Unlock'd*)

Perfumed essences were used in great quantities to scent gloves, which were a particularly popular accessory at this time.

Society men and women possessed many different pairs and some households had a resident 'glover' to cope with the enormous demand. The Earl of Bedford, who employed a glover at Woburn, had gloves scented with ambrett, jasmine and frangipane. In 1665, six pairs of gloves made for him were scented with his favourite frangipane. The Countess of Pembroke, sister of Louise de Keroualle, the king's influential French mistress, purchased 'twenty-eight pairs of open work white gloves, with orange and amber scent—the Earl of Pembroke dying, the gloves are no longer perfumed with orange and amber but violet and hyacinth'. (G. M. Crawford, *Louise de Keroualle, Duchess of Portsmouth.*) Unscented gloves were rubbed with 'jessemy butter', an aromatic ointment, and scented powder was always used on the hands before putting on gloves. An individual's taste was assessed on the choice of scent and quality of leather he used for this accessory.

> *Sir Fopling:* 'I sat near one of 'em at a Play today, and was almost Poison'd with a Pair of Cordivant Gloves he wears—'
> *Mrs. Loveit:* 'Oh! Cordivant—How I hate the smell'
> (Sir George Etherege. *The Man of Mode*)

Fashionable society at this time attached much importance to what can only be described as the trivia of fashion. During Elizabeth's reign fashion and cosmetics had been part of a broadening interest in art and colour as related to the human form. By the late seventeenth century, the attention paid to this aspect alone had grown into an absorbing obsession which, although treated in the light-hearted manner of the day, was nevertheless a time-consuming and socially important side of everyday life. 'I rise, Madam, about Ten a-clock. I don't rise sooner, because 'tis the worst thing in the World for the Complexion; not that I pretend to be a Beau; but a Man must endeavour to look wholesome, lest he make so nauseous a Figure in the Side-Bax, the Ladies shou'd be compell'd to turn their Eyes upon the Play'. (Sir John Vanbrugh, *The Relapse*.) Contemporary beaux and their ladies seemed to enjoy the same self-interest as Narcissus but, whilst he was content to admire his naturally beautiful reflection in a pool, they were intent on using every artificial aid to create their personal ideal of beauty. A total acceptance of this attitude paved the way for the most exaggerated period of artificiality in the history of English cosmetic fashions.

CHAPTER SEVEN

The Eighteenth Century

The characteristics of the Age are frenzy, folly, extravagance and insensibility (Horace Walpole)

The eighteenth century has provided a wealth of romantic material for historical novelists. The superficial picture of aristocratic society at this time is one of endless routs and soirées held in sumptiously furnished town houses. Here is a world of honourably conducted card games between 'gentlemen of quality' in fashionable gaming clubs, and of select London coffee houses where humorists indulged in a stylised repartee of wit.

The historical novelist seldom looks beyond this romantic façade of elegant town life peopled by men and women extravagantly dressed in satins, laces and powdered wigs, and with their cheeks rouged. Men and women alike wore elaborate make-up and in no other period has beauty been so artificially created. But beneath this image was often a less attractive, sometimes grotesque reality and, although an imagined ideal of natural beauty was sought after, fashion, as always, made a mockery of nature.

The eighteenth-century ideal of beauty is epitomised in portraits by Gainsborough and Reynolds (*Plate 22*). These porcelain women with powered curls and pastel silk dresses pose against a background of romanticised English countryside. The features of these society beauties are as small and perfect as those of a china doll, and their softly blushing complexions inspired the idea of the 'English Rose'.

While Gainsborough and Reynolds as fashionable portrait painters were catering to this contemporary ideal, another side of the picture can be seen through the caricatures of Thomas Rowlandson (*Plate 23*). The portrait painter panders to the vanity of his subject by eliminating imperfections and improving on reality. The caricaturist exaggerates faults and creates a vicious parody. It is difficult to know whether Gainsborough or Rowlandson painted the more truthful portraits of his contemporary subject. However, the truth is less elusive if a study is made of cosmetics used at this time. The mask of artifice that created the fashionable face was extraordinarily elaborate and recipes for eighteenth-century beauty would appal a modern cosmetologist. It needs little imagination to picture the condition of most contemporary complexions beneath the mask.

White lead still formed the main basis for cosmetics, in particular for face powder which was lavishly used by both sexes. It seems incredible that such a harmful ingredient should continue to be used. This was how white lead powder was made. 'Cast thin soft plates of lead, then roll them into shape.' Each plate was then put into a pot with a bar at the bottom to prevent the plate touching the bottom of the pot. Vinegar was then added to 'effect conversion' and finally the pots were covered with more lead plates and placed in a bed of horse manure for three weeks. After this period had elapsed, all the plates were beaten into flakes with battledores and ground into a fine powder. Water was then added and the mixture left to dry in the sun, after which it was perfumed and tinted.

The manufacture of this concoction had a significant effect on the workmen, who suffered from severe headaches, dizziness, constipation and even blindness. All these ailments were caused by the fumes of white lead. It may be imagined how much more harm was done by constant application of this powder to the sensitive skin of the face.

Inevitably, very few fashionable beauties kept their looks beyond the age of thirty. In part, this was due to an unhealthy diet and insanitary living conditions for, in spite of the outward splendour, eighteenth-century London, with open drainage and badly ventilated houses, was a breeding ground for germs. But another reason for the swift decay of beauty was the constant use of harmful cosmetics.

A case in point was that of the two famous Gunning sisters, Maria and Elizabeth, who arrived in London from Ireland in the year 1750. Their progress in society was swift, for by 1752 Elizabeth had become the Duchess of Hamilton and Maria had married the young Earl of Coventry. The sisters' elegance and classical beauty set London in an uproar. Minor poets blossomed forth in their praise:

> For ah' two Gunnings wound
> With different, yet with equal beauties crowned.

and

> their shapes are so slender, so charming their air,
> so ruddy their cheeks, their complexions so fair.

Horace Walpole was their only critic: 'these two Irish girls of no fortune, who are declared the handsomest women alive. I think their being two such handsome and both such perfect figures is their chief excellence: for singly I have seen much handsomer women than either'. But the Gunnings were the darlings of London society and, as the central attraction of every gathering, dressed and painted their faces according to fashion.

By 1760, the young Countess of Coventry was dying of consumption. Apart from the ravaging effects of disease, her beauty had faded with constant use of dangerous cosmetics.

111

Lying on her sofa with looking glass in hand, she finally asked to be carried to her bedchamber. The curtains were drawn and in a darkened room she died where none could see her pallid complexion and drawn face. Her sister, the Duchess of Hamilton, more fortunately lived to a ripe old age but her looks had also suffered by the age of thirty.

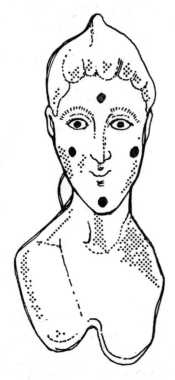

Fig 17 Salt-glazed stoneware bust of a lady wearing patches, Staffordshire, *c* 1740

There was another, more arbitrary reason for early loss of beauty. Smallpox, that widespread scourge, left faces pitted and marked for life. It was the disfiguring effects of this disease which had been instrumental in starting the fashion of applying patches to the face, the ideal camouflage for pock marks. The patch, or *mouche*, was in common use in the eighteenth

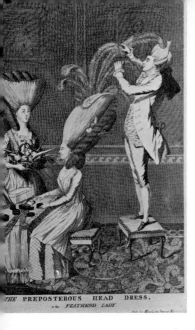

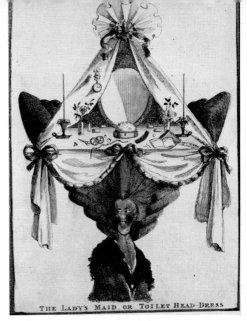

THE PREPOSTEROUS HEAD DRESS,
or the FEATHERD LADY

THE LADY'S MAID, OR TOILET HEAD-DRESS

bove left) 'The Prepostrous Headdress of the Feathered Lady'. A satirical view of a
mporary hairstyle. Powdered wigs were generally worn, but many women had their
uilt up into a mountain of curls with the aid of false hair pieces. The finished article
bled an exotic gateau.

bove right) 'The Lady's Maid, or Toilet Head-dress'. An amusing fantasy illustration
ning the exaggerated hairstyle of the day with a representation of a contemporary
ng table.

low) The Countess's Morning Levee, from William Hogarth's 'Marriage á la Mode'.
ociety lady's elaborate *toilette* took so long to complete that guests were entertained
while, so that no time was wasted away from the social scene.

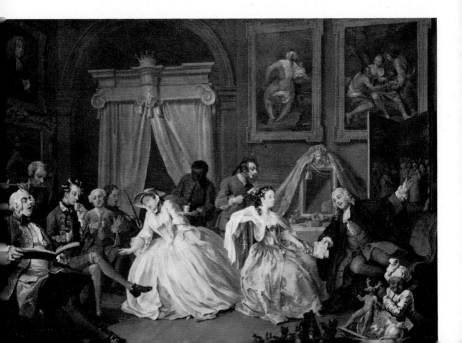

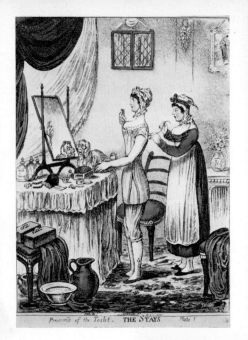

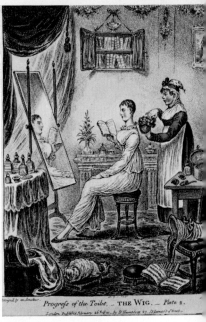

Progress of the Toilet. THE STAYS. *Plate 1.*

Progress of the Toilet. — THE WIG. — *Plate 2.*

London. Pub.d Feb.y 26 1810 by H. Humphrey 27. St James's Street.

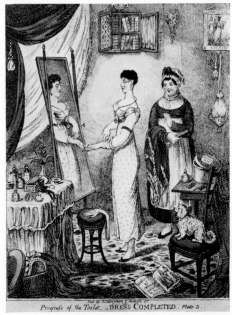

Progress of the Toilet. — DRESS COMPLETED. *Plate 3.*

27 'The Progress of the Toilet' by James Gillray. A series of satirical illustrations sh[ow]
three stages of a Regency lady's toilet: 'The Stays', 'The Wig' and 'The Dress Compl[eted]'
with particular interesting detail of the contemporary dressing room and toilet table.

century. Cut out of silk, taffeta or even Spanish leather, it was variously shaped and coloured; black was popular, with bright scarlet a close favourite.

Those who were seriously disfigured by smallpox patched their faces to such an extent that Steele (Isaac Bickerstaff), of *The Tatler*, writes to a female correspondent with a concern owing more to aesthetics than gallantry:

> Madam,
> Let me beg of you to take off the patches at the lower end of your left cheek and I will allow two more under your left eye, which will contribute more to the symmetry of your face; except you would please to remove the ten black atoms on your Ladyship's chin, and wear one large patch instead of them. If so, you may properly enough retain the three patches above mentioned.
>
> I am etc.

As Steele indicates, this fashion was not an exclusively feminine one. 'There lay a Male Coquet. He had a bottle of salts hanging over his Head, and upon the table by his bedside, Suckling's poems, with a little heap of black patches on it.'

Eighteenth-century society must have been grateful for this bizarre fashion as most skins were blemished by pock marks. The only women reputed to retain a perfect complexion were milkmaids, who were immunised from smallpox by catching a mild form of the disease from cattle. This gave rise to the popular nursery rhyme:

> Where are you going to my pretty maid
> I'm going a-milking, Sir, she said

and

> What is your fortune my pretty maid
> My face is my fortune, Sir, she said.

Lady Wortley Montagu, an unusual woman of great personality, had been disfigured in her youth by smallpox. Against opposition, she campaigned persistently for inoculation and

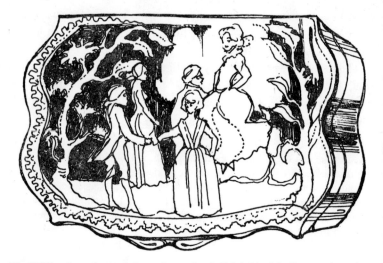

Fig 18 Piqué-work patch box of tortoiseshell inlaid with silver and mother-of-pearl, French, *c* 1740

had the courage to allow her beloved son to be the first person in England to be immunised in this way. By the end of the century, in spite of warnings from sceptical diehards and cynics, her efforts were rewarded. Many people were inoculated and patches were less frequently worn.

Mouseskin eyebrows were another false 'additive' to beauty. Men and women trimmed and tortured their own eyebrows into shape, blackening them with lead combs, but fashion dictated that this was no substitute for elegant artificial brows. Unfortunately, these did not always stay in place, and it was a familiar sight to see frantic adjustments being made with an air of apparently unconcerned nonchalance.

In an age when even the fashionable relied on an unhealthy diet, teeth soon rotted and discoloured. A false porcelain set proved a popular camouflage and 'plumpers' were used to swell sunken cheeks to a fashionable roundness. 'Plumpers' were small cork balls worn inside the cheeks and, with the additional impediment of false teeth, many an individual became tongue-tied and silent. Inevitably, 'plumpers' did much to contribute to the fashionable lisp, so desirable amongst ladies of society.

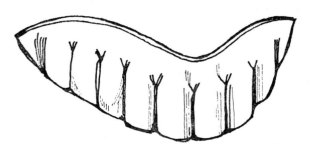

Fig 19 Solid carved-ivory false teeth for upper jaw, eighteenth or early nineteenth century

An amalgam of all these items of cosmetic artifice gives a clear picture of the appearance of eighteenth-century men and women. Their faces were painted porcelain-white with lead powder, their eyebrows supplemented with mouseskin and their cheeks dotted with patches and rounded with 'plumpers'. Rouge added the finishing touch to the fashionable complexion.

Rouges included carmine; *rouge blanche* made from a white lead base, as the name implies; 'vegetable rouge' which suggests a vegetable dye, and 'serviette rouge', a rag dipped in colouring dye. Rouge, apart from 'serviette rouge', was applied with Spanish or Chinese wool and was considered to be the most vital part of face make-up: 'The last box of rouge he sent me was too pale by at least two tinges—and you know Sir Harry, there is no making a decent complexion, unless the rouge is in perfection.' ('The Macaroni Dialogue', *Ladies Magazine*, 1773.)

Lips were also rouged with carmine or painted with lipsticks, which were made from ground plaster of Paris, with colouring added according to choice.

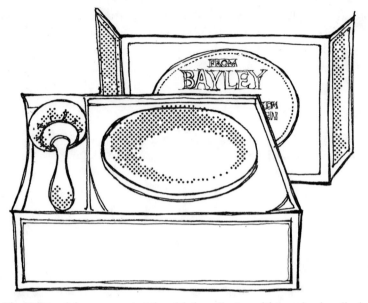

Fig 20 Porcelain rouge pot and padded applicator with wooden handle, in original cardboard box labelled 'From Bayley and Blew, Cockspur Street, London', late eighteenth century

Once the full range of cosmetics had been bestowed on the face, it remained to attend to the hair. Powdered wigs were generally worn, but many women had their own hair built up into a mountain of curls with the aid of false hair pieces (*Plate 24*). The finished article, which resembled an exotic gâteau, was liberally dusted with white powder and decorated with feathers and artificial flowers. The most adept of lady's maids took so long to dress these coiffures that the time set aside for the completion of the *toilette* would have been excessive. Rather than commit a social blunder, many women had their hair set, so to speak, to last over a period of weeks or even a month.

The 'set' consisted of holding the hair together with lard, which undoubtedly went rancid after a day, let alone a month.

It was hardly surprising that hair became verminous, as did wigs, which were seldom cleaned. To relieve irritation, a narrow pronged stick of ivory was specially designed for the purpose of scratching the scalp. Unfortunately, not only did this disturb the fleas but also mice, which were frequently found nesting in the hair. To prevent mice or rats attacking the larded hair, nightcaps of silver or gold wire were sometimes worn at bedtime. This practice must have proved just as drastic a defence of the lady's chastity as any belt invented by a medieval knight.

Having dealt with her basic *toilette* of face make-up and hairstyle, the eighteenth-century woman would then have dressed suitably for the day's social engagements. It only remained to choose some exotic perfume to accord with the mood of the dress, and the *toilette* was complete.

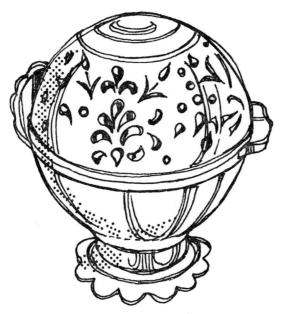

Fig 21 Brass soap box with pierced decoration, English, eighteenth century

117

Perfume was used liberally by both sexes, and much care went into the choice of the right scent for an occasion. French perfumes were as popular as they are today. The English House of Yardley had a flourishing soap and perfumery business in London and their famous lavender water was already a favourite. Hungary water was another *eau de toilette* that was often used; a contemporary recipe for this includes rosemary oil, verbena oil, Portugal oil, linette oil, peppermint oil, triple rose water, triple orange flower water and ninety per cent alchohol.

Apart from its obviously delightful qualities, perfume was an essential deodorant in the eighteenth century. The lavish and elaborate clothing was virtually impossible to clean, so perfumed sachets were sewn into the linings to ensure a degree of freshness. Since contemporary perfumes had none of the lasting fragrance of modern scents, this proved an ineffective measure and stale perfume contributed to the unpleasant odour of unclean garments.

A general lack of bathing was another reason for the liberal use of perfume. Bathrooms were not unknown, but they were merely status symbols. Sporting a truly magnificent outward show of silk curtains, the bathroom usually contained nothing but a redundant wooden bath tub.

Thus, in a world where men and women possessed none of our standards of hygiene, dirt and odour were disguised by renewed applications of perfume, and bad skins were camouflaged by a cosmetic mask of potentially dangerous materials. There was some attempt to improve the standards of hygiene in cosmetics in 1724, when an act was passed to ensure a careful examination of drugs. Some preparations became safer to use, but many people still preferred the old harsh, white lead paints.

Some advertisements, however, stressed the medicinal properties in make-up, proving that there was a market for cosmetics which contributed to skin improvement:

118

This Chrystal Cosmetick, approved of by the worthy Dr. Paul Chamberline, viz. by washing Morning or Evening, cures all red faces, proceeding from what cause, forever takes off all Morphew, Pimples, and Freckles; it is of a Soft Nature, cleansing and adorning the Face and Hands of both sexes in a very beautiful manner and may be used with as much safety as milk, having in it no Mercury (so frequently made use of). Price of the largest Bottle 6s. the lesser 3s. Sold at Mr. Alcrofts by Exchange Alley, Cornhill. Mr. Jackson's the corner of Wood Street, Cheapside. Mrs. Brecknocks, the Upper end of St. James' Street, Piccadilly. To prevent counterfeits each single bottle, with directions, is tied and sealed with this Coat of Arms a Frett with a Lion rampart in a Canton (*The Tatler*)

A second advertisement deals with the hands:

A most incomparable Paste for the Hands far exceeding anything ever yet in print it makes them most delicately white, slick and plump, fortifies them against the sharpness of the Air, or Scorching of the Fire; A Hand cannot be so spoiled, but the constant use of this Paste will recover it; Sold only at Mr. Alcrofts Toyshop over-against the Royal Exchange at 1s. 6d. the Pot with Directions (*The Tatler*)

The wording of these advertisements suggests the exaggerations of a fairground doctor, but this did not deter people from believing in the miracle cure with its promises of procuring beauty in a bottle. The hopeful belief in an instant remedy for pimples and spots has always been a human failing and explains the success of many charlatans in the field of beauty.

Giuseppe Balsamo, who called himself the Count Alessandro Cagliostro, was just such a man. He arrived in London from the Continent in 1771 and bought a house in Whitcomb Street where he established his laboratory. Alchemy was his speciality, but he also manufactured love potions, cosmetics and his famous water of life, which he claimed preserved youth and beauty for ever.

119

Charm with women helped him to sell his concoctions and he possessed the added attraction of an aura of mystery surrounding his life. An experienced medium, he dabbled in witchcraft and astrology, all of which endeared him to the female sex who believed that by purchasing his lotions and ointments they were acquiring a magical recipe for beauty.

Cagliostro's products were excessively expensive, as were many cosmetics at this time. Prices went up still further in 1786 when a heavy purchase tax was imposed on all cosmetics and shops retailing this commodity had to have a special licence.

A sense of economy undoubtedly prompted many to manufacture cosmetics at home, although, judging by contemporary women's magazines, the invention of recipes for beauty was a common art throughout this century. The ingredients used would often have been more at home in a witch's cauldron. Frog's blood, leeches and goat's grease sound like preparations for a coven feast rather than for a compound in aid of beauty. But there were no lengths to which an eighteenth-century woman would not go to make herself beautiful enough to attract a husband or lover. Men also believed that much could be achieved by cosmetic perfection, although an amusing letter in the *Gentleman's Magazine* of 1773 discredits this belief: 'I dress fashionably and therefore wear a great deal of powder.' The correspondent goes on to explain that whilst visiting his love of the moment, who has just lost her father, her mother walks into the room to discover the two lovers sitting together on the sofa. Her daughter's 'black silk gown, curse on the mourning' is 'whiter than ordinary and guessing we have been closer than we then were, she civilly desired me to walk down'.

Although extravagances in cosmetic fashions were frequently ridiculed by members of society who were unwilling to spend time in titivation, the majority of men and women continued to indulge in every form of cosmetic artifice. As new ointments and lotions were invented, so they were purchased, adding to an ever-growing collection of pots, bottles, powders and paints. It can be imagined that the average dressing table was littered with cosmetic paraphernalia. There were jars of pomade and rouge, pots of face and hair powder, crystal scent bottles and enamelled patch boxes, a variety of home-made ointments, and exotic cosmetic concoctions made with drugs and spices imported from Baghdad, Turkey, Cyprus, Spain, Italy and France (*Plate 25*). French cosmetics were considered the finest and no dressing table was complete without a collection of Parisian paints and powders.

A spoof advertisement for the recovery of stolen goods, in the November 1710 issue of *The Tatler*, lists the contents of a dressing table:

> Seven cakes of superfine Spanish Wool, Two pairs of bran-new plumpers, Four black-lead combs, Three pairs of fashionable Eyebrows, Two sets of ivory teeth (little the worse for wearing), and a collection of Receipts to make Pastes for the Hands, Pomatums, Lip Salves, white pots, Beautifying creams, Water of Talc and Frog Spawn water and Decoctions for cleaning the complexion.

This cosmetic equipment was undoubtedly typical of every boudoir in town, but Alexander Pope gives a more romantic image of the eighteenth-century boudoir in 'The Rape of the Lock':

> And all Arabia breathes from yonder box
> The tortoise here and elephant unite
> Transformed to combs, the speckled and the white
> Here files of Pins extend their shining Rows,
> Puffs, Powders, Patches, Bibles, Billet Doux.

The application of the entire fashionable cosmetic paraphernalia was, as may be imagined, a lengthy process: 'My hours of existence, on being awake are from eleven in the morning to eleven at night, half of which I leave to myself, in picking my teeth, washing my hands, pairing my nails and looking in the glass.' (*The Tatler*, 1709.) Thus it became necessary to entertain guests during the arrangement of one's *toilette* for, in this way, no time was wasted away from the social scene (*Plate 26*). The latest love affairs, duels and scandals could be discussed whilst adjusting a patch on the cheek or powdering some extravagant coiffure.

In a social world where so much time was spent in personal adornment, dress and cosmetic fashions acquired an exaggerated importance. This prompted a group of young men to form a club whose identity depended on the way its members dressed. The 'Macaroni Club' drew its membership from the youthful élite who had done the Grand Tour of Europe; a passing flirtation with Italian culture had given them the intellectual conceit of most dilettantes. Walpole comments, 'the Macaroni Club is composed of all the travelled young men who wear long curls and spying glasses'.

The 'Macaronis' set new fashions in dress and make-up, and in their use of cosmetics they made an artifice out of artifice. The elaborate care taken over the exact placing of a patch, rouging of a cheek or tinting of a powder made the 'Macaroni' a joke amongst members of society who could laugh at the follies of fashion. He was ridiculed in such farcical skits as 'The Macaroni Dialogue' which appeared in the *Ladies Magazine*. Sir Harry Dimple, the central character, declaims, 'It was me that first improved upon the Poudre à la Maréchale and by throwing in a dash of the violet, brought it to such high perfection, you may always distinguish me by the peculiar odouriferousness of my powder.' In another issue of the *Ladies Magazine*, a 'Macaroni' is sarcastically described as 'A thing that has some resemblance to a man' but who 'Holds his Head up, wears his hair powdered and curled, and never goes out till he has formed his countenance according to the rules of the latest fashion.'

'Macaroni' became used to describe any man or woman who made a fetish of their toilet. 'Methinks one of these Macaronis of the sex, if she is capable of thinking, must be cruelly mortified on approaching to her toilette. On seeing her tête, her pomade, her rouge, her patch box, etc. She can hardly help saying to herself—there is my beauty—my complexion is in that box.' (*Ladies Magazine*, 1773.)

The *Ladies Magazine* was a vehicle for puritan opinions, but it is obvious that it merely voiced many of the feelings of its readers. In every age of extravagant fashions and excessive artifice, there is an underlying movement to restore balance and a true sense of values. The *Ladies Magazine* constantly advocates that 'Natural Beauty, the agremens of dress, mental abilities and virtues are the sources of pleasing'.

In the early part of the eighteenth century, fashionable society paid no attention to these prudish dictates, as dress and cosmetics were a great source of enjoyment, but towards the end of the century there was a swing back to puritan ideals. Young fops and their feminine counterparts were ridiculed and criticised:

> They have been told a thousand times that white robs their face of its expression and that rouge made that bloom and freshness of complexion disappear . . . They illuminate themselves after the manner of the ancient Bacchanalians and render their eyes more piercing. This custom which was in use among the most savage nations transforms the prettiest face into a painted pagoda (*Ladies' Magazine*, 1773)

The puritan movement had many champions, including Alexander Pope who described fashionable society earlier in the century as:

> Such painted Puppets, such a varnish'd Race
> Of hollow Gewgaws, only Dress and Face
> ('Satires of Dr John Donne')

This harsh criticism was echoed by many people in the latter half of the century and proof of the general revulsion against all artifice is provided by the passing of an extraordinary act of parliament in the year 1770. It was expressly designed to protect men beguiled into marriage by the false adornments of the female 'Macaroni':

> All women, of whatever age, rank, profession, or degree, whether virgins, maids, or widows, that shall, from and after such Act, impose upon, seduce, and betray into matrimony, any of his Majesty's subjects, by the scents, paints, cosmetic washes, artificial teeth, false hair, Spanish wool, iron stays, hoops, high-heeled shoes and bolstered hips, shall incur the penalty of the law in force against witchcraft and like misdemeanours and that the marriage, upon conviction, shall stand null and void.

There is no evidence that this act has ever been repealed.

The writings of such men as Rousseau had influenced society to turn away from the excesses of fashion to a simpler way of life. This movement was precipitated further by the French Revolution of 1789 which marked the end of aristocratic society in France. Paris, with its artificial, urbanised way of life, had set the pattern for London society but, with the Revolution, this influence ceased to exist. The English, who have always had a deep love of the country, spent more time on their estates, and town was no longer the centre of society life.

Fashions in dress and make-up were influenced by this change of social scene, and the rouges, paints and powders which had earlier seemed so attractive were now considered vulgar. Face powder was chiefly applied to the neck. The extravagant confections of powdered curls had disappeared in favour of softer hairstyles which remained unpowdered. Rouge was out of fashion, and 'patching' had lost its purpose with the increasingly successful results of smallpox inoculation. Horace Walpole, describing a group of contemporary young men, writes, 'It seems they now crop their hair short and wear no powder.'

124

The artificial hothouse existence of mid-eighteenth century London, with its fops and painted ladies, was at an end. An anonymous contributor to the *Gentlemen's Magazine* writes what could be taken for an epitaph of the passing age:

> Dress and paint then lay aside
> Of borrowed Beauty leave the Pride
> Studied Art and Vain Disguise
> Men admire not but Despise.

CHAPTER EIGHT

The Nineteenth Century

Make a hole in a lemon, fill it with sugar candy, and close it nicely with leaf gold, applied over the rind that was cut out; then roast the lemon in hot ashes. When desirous of using the juice, squeeze out a little through the hole already made, and wash the face with a napkin wetted therewith. This juice is said to cleanse the skin and brighten the complexion marvellously.

(Anon. *The Art of Beauty*, 1825)

The decline of extravagance in dress and cosmetic fashions continued during the last years of the eighteenth century and a new style of appearance evolved which heralded a return to elegance. The painted beauties of the previous age would have had little success in winning praise from the lips of a sophisticated Regency gentleman.

The new ideal of feminine beauty is illustrated by the fashion plates of the day. A powdered *coiffure* had disappeared in favour of softly coiled black hair embellished with tendrils of ringlets on the cheeks; large dark eyes added expressive emphasis to a pale-complexioned face with delicately formed piquant features (*Plates 27, 29*). The society woman, clothed in her high-waisted dress of soft fabric, appeared light-boned and pretty, acting as a perfect foil for the handsome masculinity of her escort.

An elegant appearance became essential to the 'gentleman of fashion' and this was undoubtedly due to the influence of Beau Brummell (*Plate 28*). Misleadingly described as a prince of dandies, his taste, far from being flamboyant, was distinctive because of its restraint. His style of dress depended on the simplicity of plain dark cloth superbly cut and tailored to fit the figure and his immaculately groomed appearance owed nothing to artifice but everything to his insistence on scrupulous cleanliness. Brummell never used cosmetic paints on his face, but immersed it in fresh water every morning, alternately scrubbing and rinsing it to tone up the complexion. Following his example, many society men abandoned even the slightest hint of powder or rouge and, although a few painted dandies still walked furtively down Bond Street, they were exceptions to the general rule.

Brummell's *toilette* was the subject of endless gossip and many of these stories were spread round town by Brummell himself. It was rumoured that he sent all his laundry to the country so that when his linen returned to London it was scented by the fresh smell of fields and flowers. He was reputed to shave his face several times and pluck out any remaining hairs with tweezers. He employed three hairdressers: 'The first is responsible for my temples, the second for the front and the third for the occiput.'

He was a notable influence on the Prince Regent whose taste in heavy flower perfumes changed to the use of a light cologne favoured by Brummell. As a result delicate scents became fashionable and therefore the unpleasant odour of an unwashed body could no longer be camouflaged by the aroma of a strong perfume. This encouraged bathing as a regular daily habit, although many members of society still regarded cleanliness with suspicion. The elderly Duke of Norfolk could only be washed when he was too drunk to be aware of the experience.

Hair had also to be cleaned more frequently as powder was no longer used to disguise a dirty head. A powdered *coiffure* had become unfashionable since the French Revolution and Brummell is reputed to have bought himself out of the army

because officers were still expected to whiten their curls artificially. Pitt's heavy tax on hair powder also contributed to the
end of this fashion, although Lord William Murray, son of the
Duke of Atholl, attempted to evade the tax by taking out a
patent to manufacture powder from horse chestnuts. Society
men of the day were so determined to avoid taxation that they
ceased to wear their hair long, tied back and powdered. 'Such
is the universal disgust at the powder tax, that many thousands
of the male sex have already sacrificed their favorite curls to
disappoint the rapacity of a minister'. ('Peter Pindar', 1816.)
The tax was also extremely unpopular with women who still
hankered after the unfashionable whitened *coiffures* of a past
age:

> Lo, the poor girl, whom carrot-colour shocks,
> Pines pennyless, and blushes for her locks.
> Refus'd to fly to powder's friendly aid,
> She bids them seek in caps the secret shade;
> No ringlets now around her neck to wave,
> Phillis must hid the redd'ning shame or shave!
> At thee she flings her curses, Pitt, and cries—
> At thee she darts the lightnings of her eyes;
> And thinks that love ne'er warm'd him who could vex
> With wanton strokes of cruelty, the sex.
>
> ('Peter Pindar')

The lack of powdered curls, however, was responsible for
the charming appearance of Regency ladies, and the natural
locks favoured by men also became fashionable for women.
This aversion for artifice was to continue through most of
the nineteenth century and, although a sparing use of powder
and rouge may have enhanced the complexion, brightly coloured
dyes were considered vulgar.

Cosmetics made from herbs, flowers, vegetable fats and oils
replaced those harmful concoctions of the eighteenth century,
which had attempted to disguise a defective skin under a thick

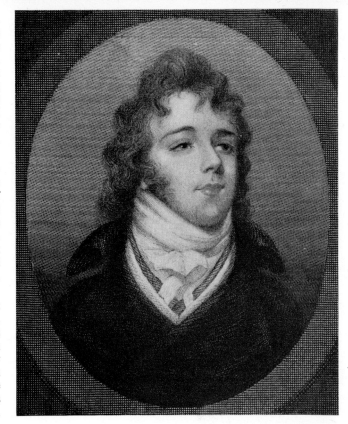

(*right*) Beau Brummell. Engraving from a portrait miniature. Brummell's style of appearance, which depended on immaculate grooming and scrupulous cleanliness, was copied by every Regency gentleman of fashion.

(*below left*) Regency fashion plate. The contemporary ideal of beauty was far removed from that of the eighteenth-century. Dark-haired women with lively, piquant, natural looks were favoured.

(*below right*) A lady at the court of St James. Head and shoulders detail. The Victorian ideal of femininity depended on an untouched, childlike appearance, soft ringlets and a virtuous manner.

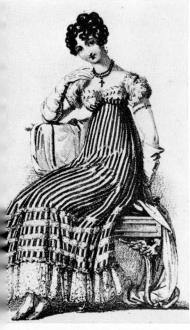

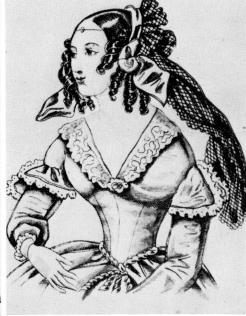

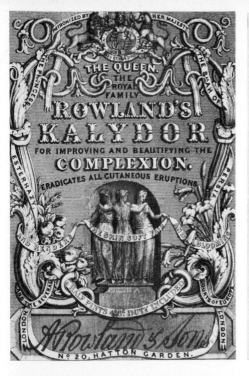

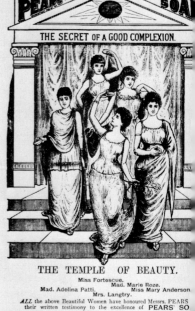

THE TEMPLE OF BEAUTY.

Miss Fortescue.
Mad. Marie Roze.
Mad. Adelina Patti. Miss Mary Anderson
Mrs. Langtry.

ALL the above Beautiful Women have honoured Messrs. PEARS
their written testimony to the excellence of PEARS' SO
FOR IMPROVING THE HANDS AND COMPLEXION

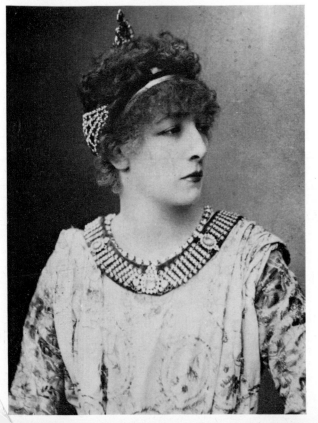

31 (*above left*) Label fo
Rowland's 'Kalydor fo
Improving and Beautif
the Complexion'.

32 (*above right*) Advert
leaflet for Pears' soap.
illustration showing se
well-known beauties o
day, including Lily La
issuing from the 'Temp
Beauty'. Pears were we
ahead of their time wit
ideas on advertising.

33 (*left*) Sarah Bernhar
Famous actress and be
whose profile Oscar W
likened to that on a R
coin, she used a kohl-l
make-up to emphasise
eyes and a great deal o
white face powder. Sh
rouged her lips in publi
habit almost unprecede
in the 1880s.

mask of paint, and this emphasis on natural ingredients encouraged the art of home-made beauty. As a result many books
were written at this period, inviting the housewife to manufacture her own toilet preparations. A good example of one of
these works was *The Art of Beauty*. Published anonymously in
1825, during George IV's reign, it illustrates the new approach
to cosmetics which aimed at improving the natural condition
of the skin instead of artificially camouflaging its faults.

Stress is laid on the importance of cleanliness: 'Bathing along
with friction is an essential part of beauty-training, for clearing
the skin of its impurities, and giving transparency and freshness
to the complexion.' Steam baths were particularly recommended for this purpose and the anonymous writer's recipe for
one of these, using steaming kettles, pipes and a large blanket,
would have inspired Heath Robinson.

A variety of lotions, ointments, washes and salves were
suggested for use after bathing and these all purported to
enhance the true beauty of a natural complexion. A pale skin
was still fashionable so that many of the recipes were designed
to prevent sunburn or erase freckles; these concoctions were
made from such ingredients as horse radish, sour milk, rain
water, lavender and appetizing mixtures of cream, sugar, lemon
and grapes.

Although the book states that 'When a person is young, and
fresh, and handsome, to paint would be perfectly ridiculous',
the writer grudgingly admits that 'art can often perform
wonders, which could not, by the uninitiated, be conceived to
be within the limits of possibility'. Thus, a subtle rouge was
recommended for use on the face, but lip colouring was
obviously considered undesirable and vulgar. Vegetable rouges
made from red sandalwood, cochineal, brazil wood and saffron
mixed with talc powder were favoured, instead of red lead dyes
which contained sulphur and mercury, and home-made preparations were considered preferable to purchased concoctions.

Exceptions were 'Portuguese rouge', contained in china dishes and only genuine if imported from Portugal; 'Spanish wool', in cakes about 'the size and thickness of a crown-piece', the best variety of which was manufactured by Jews in London, and 'Spanish papers', which misleadingly came from China. 'Chinese Boxes of colours' were also considered safe and harmless, and they were possibly the first examples of 'make-up palettes' to be found in England. These japanned boxes contained twenty-four papers each enveloping three smaller papers, one for the eyebrows, impregnated with a black substance; another for rouging the cheeks, and lastly a paper containing half an ounce of white powder made from ground pearls.

Pearl white was extremely popular at this period, and talc, which had replaced white lead as a face blanche, was considered an excellent alternative. The toxic properties of metallic-based paints had finally been discovered through the advances made in chemical analysis, but the author of *The Art of Beauty* nevertheless warned his readers that home-made powder was safer than any which could be bought in the shops.

The patience of the home beautician must have been prodigious, as she was expected to manufacture her own dentifrices and mouth washes, eye lotions, lip salves and even depilatories.

Depilatory Vegetable Essence

Take polypody of the oak, cut into very small pieces, and put a quantity into a glass cucurbit. Pour on this as much Lisbon or French white wine as will rise an inch above the ingredients, and digest it in a hot water or vapour bath for twenty four hours.

An alternative recipe suggests that 'the distilled water of the leaves and roots of celandine, is said to have a similar effect; and likewise, oil of walnuts'.

Hair pomades, oils, cleansers and dyes occupy an important place among cosmetic recipes, and many of these preparations seem to be based on the ancient natural remedies of the Middle Ages and Elizabethan England. 'Lye', made from ashes, was recommended as a 'shampoo', bear's grease as a pomade, and juice of nettles and herbs as a conditioner. A hair bleach suggested the use of 'a quart of lye prepared from the ashes of vine-twigs, briony, celandine-roots, and turmeric, of each half an ounce; saffron and lily-roots, of each two drachms; flowers of mullein, yellow stechas, broom and St John's Wort, of each a drachm'. (*The Art of Beauty.*)

The home-made cosmetic continued to be the main aid to beauty when Queen Victoria ascended the throne in 1837 and numerous books on the subject were published during her reign. The increasing number of women's journals supplied their readers with toiletry recipes and articles on beauty, which were sandwiched between household hints on how to make Scotch marmalade or wash cotton, and romantic stories and poems entitled 'The Midshipman's Farewell' and 'The Soul's Ideal'.

However, the Victorian image of feminine beauty demanded less of cosmetics, whether home-made or purchased, than ever before; by comparison, the ladies of Regency and Georgian England were positively liberal in their use of toilet preparations. The perfect Victorian woman is idealised in the fashion prints of the day and described in contemporary novels (*Plate 30*). She possessed the innocent face of a china doll, with a rosebud mouth, dimpled cheeks and small neat features framed by a demure hairstyle of ringlets. Charles Dickens' description of David Copperfield's child bride, Dora, with her ingenuous manner, her blushes and curls, would have won the heart of any Victorian man: 'I never saw such curls—how could I, for there never were such curls!—as those she shook out to hide her blushes'.

The preference for a child-like, untouched prettiness meant that women had to resort to subterfuge if they wished to use cosmetics which artificially coloured their complexions. Rouge

131

and powder were applied so sparingly, with a hare's foot or a camel hair brush, that they could scarcely be noticed; and lip salves, which cunningly concealed a touch of carmine, could only be used with the excuse of moistening chapped lips.

Washing with soap and hot water was now thought to be the best aid to beauty that any woman needed to improve her appearance, and there is no doubt that in Victorian England cleanliness was considered a virtue second only to godliness. Daily bathing became an established routine in upper and middle class households, and although bathrooms, as such, only made their appearance towards the end of the century, hip baths in the bedroom were an adequate alternative which even Queen Victoria made use of in Buckingham Palace.

The fetish for cleanliness led to the construction of public baths and wash houses, provided with hot and cold water; the city of Liverpool built the first of its kind in England in 1842. In 1846 parliament passed an act encouraging other cities to follow this example and also providing a scale of approved charges for the poor and higher income groups, which indicates that these baths were for general use.

As a further aid to cleanliness, the manufacture of soaps had become a thriving industry in Victorian England and, once the heavy tax of threepence on every pound of soap had been halved in 1833 and repealed by Gladstone twenty years later, everybody could afford to buy it. By the middle of the century there were factories in London, Liverpool, Bristol and other cities and approximately 136 million lb of soap were manufactured every year. This article of toiletry had a special section devoted to it at the Great Exhibition of 1851; in spite of foreign competition, British soaps won seven of the prize medals, and Yardley and Statham acquired an honourable mention for their Old Brown Windsor soap. The excellent reputation which English manufacturers enjoyed abroad led to the adoption of the brand name 'Windsor Soap' by many foreign factories,

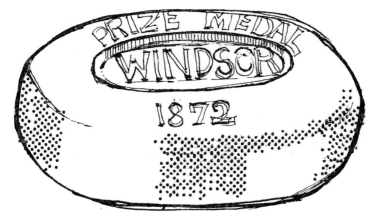

Fig 22 Prize-winning 'Windsor' soap, English, nineteenth century

including a Polish firm who used it for their finest quality product.

Perfumery also occupied an important place at the Great Exhibition. The English firm, Gibbs, introduced the first perfumed toilet soap and British manufacturers won two prize medals for their scents and one for artificial essences. Foreign exhibitors came from all over the world; there were displays of exotic scents from the Middle East and sophisticated perfumes from France, while John Maria Farina's *cologne* was exhibited by means of a spectacular fountain. Parisian scents were considered the finest and won many prizes, including an honourable mention for the perfumery of Eugene Rimmel, a

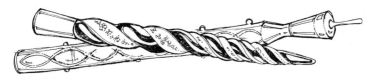

Fig 23 'Oxford Lavender' scent bottles of gilt and enamel decoration, imported from Europe in large quantities during the nineteenth century

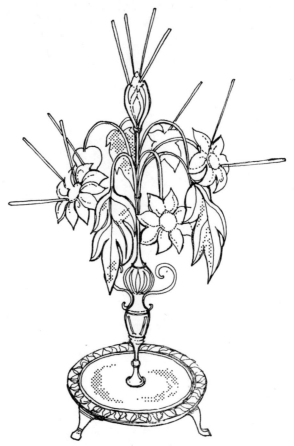

Fig 24 Silver toothpick holder, Portuguese, *c* 1853–61

man whose name was to become famous in the cosmetic industry. English perfumiers could not compete with those of the Continent and, although as a light scent Yardley's lavender water enjoyed a good reputation abroad, France produced a much greater variety of perfumes.

In 1855, in his book *The Art of Perfumery*, a chemist named Septimus Piesse tried to revolutionise the English perfume

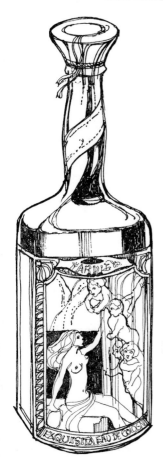

Fig 25 'Exquisita' eau de cologne bottle, English, late nineteenth century

industry. He wrote appealing to British horticulturists and perfumiers to unite their expertise in an effort to loosen the French hold on the market. With all the commercial optimism of the true Victorian, he suggested that the vast resources of the Empire could be employed to contribute to this enterprise. Many of the colonies had ideal temperatures and climates for the cultivation of flowers, and they also had natural sources of ingredients which could be used in the manufacture of scent.

135

He had already encouraged his brother Charles, colonial secretary for Western Australia, to establish flower farms in this region, but his brother's death and a general lack of confidence in his enterprising ideas meant that unfortunately they never came to fruition.

The Victorian sense of commercial adventure and the increasing respectability of trade encouraged the growth of advertising. Numerous advertisements for toilet preparations were carried by magazines and also began to appear on posters. In 1888, Pears created a sensation by purchasing 'Bubbles', the famous painting by Millais, for reproduction as a poster to advertise their soap, and other soap manufacturers, like Sunlight, swiftly followed this example by employing the talents of well-known artists for their advertisements. But the most persistent advertisers of toiletry throughout the century were Rowlands, whose Kalydor and Macassar oil enjoyed nation-wide popularity (*Plates 31, 32*).

Macassar oil was chiefly employed by men to dress their hair and it led to the design of anti-macassar cloths for the backs of chairs to protect upholstery from grease stains. Home-made recipes for this pomade were numerous and the unfortunate housewife was obviously expected to concoct toilet preparations for her husband as well as for herself. Shaving soaps and after-shave lotions with such pleasant sounding names as 'Cherry Laurel Water' fill the pages of 'home beauty' books, evidence that the Victorian man was very particular about his personal grooming. Dandies of the age prided themselves on their luxuriant moustaches or elegant beards. They even on occasion used hair dyes. Disraeli is known to have dyed his hair and he is believed to have commented on the fact that Lords Malmesbury, Palmerston and Lyndhurst employed rouge to embellish their appearance. This practice was reputed to be not uncommon among high-ranking army officers, who were notorious dandies.

136

Although the Victorian man could blatantly use cosmetic devices, women of the day had to disguise any attempts at self-improvement. The prudery of contemporary moral standards was totally prohibitive as far as female vanity was concerned, but in spite of these restrictions many women attempted to find secret ways of improving on nature.

The need for absolute secrecy in the pursuit of beauty explains the success of an extraordinary charlatan, Sarah Rachel Leverson, who traded under the name of 'Madame Rachel'. In 1863 she opened her salon at 47a, New Bond Street, with the inviting legend 'Beautiful For Ever' displayed above the door. Although this brazen approach to beauty indicated a certain lack of delicacy, her customers were assured of her complete discretion in guarding their identity from any publicity. Her advertising manifesto was dramatically worded: 'Beautiful for ever! Yes, beautiful for ever! Lovely as the bright sunshine at morning's dawn, beautiful as the dew-drops on the flowers, so beautiful is lovely Woman! . . . Who has shown the civilized world, and the greatest nation of it, how wise and good has ever been the influence of beautiful Woman? Our glorious and beloved Queen, who bright and beautiful, came forth to the nation in her young and lovely girlhood'. However, her praises for womankind's natural virtues and beauty become tempered with such remarks as, 'How frequently we find that a slight blemish on the face, otherwise divinely beautiful, has occasioned a sad and solitary life of celibacy—unloved, unblessed and ultimately unwept and unremembered'. But she assures her readers that her expertise as a beautician and consultant to the Sultana of Turkey will render them immune from this unfortunate end.

Her cosmetics were so prohibitively expensive that only women with a substantial purse could afford her prices. These preparations had exotic names, such as 'Circassian Beauty Wash', 'Armenian Liquid for Removing Wrinkles', 'Favorite of the Harem's Pearl White', 'Chinese Leaves for the Cheeks and Lips', 'Magnetic Rock Dew Water of the Sahara' and 'Senses of Peace', and they were priced at one to two guineas a container. Madame Rachel's scale of charges rose abruptly with the sale of 'Jordan Water' and 'Venus's Toilet', each costing ten to twenty guineas per bottle, and reached its peak with 'The Royal Arabian Toilet of Beauty', a course of baths priced at one hundred to a thousand guineas. Although her cosmetics purported to be made from rare herbs and ingredients imported from the East, the materials used for their manufacture were of humble origins and the famous Arabian baths consisted of a mixture of bran and hot water.

The end of Madame Rachel's career was in sight when she resorted to blackmailing the widow of an Indian army officer into paying the large sum of £1,400. The ensuing court case took the country by storm, as the national Press devoted a great deal of space to the legal proceedings which, judging from the transcript of the trial, were frequently hilariously amusing. They also aroused a fiercely righteous indignation in the contemporary public, who were no doubt delighted when Madame Rachel received the heavy sentence of five years' penal servitude.

Although beauty establishments were thrown into disrepute by this infamous charlatan, in 1886 Mrs Frances Hemming opened a salon in London which sold her toilet preparations under the brand name of Cyclax. Her cosmetics were expensive, but their fine quality gained her an exclusive clientele, who arrived discreetly veiled in their carriages at the door of the salon and were ushered in secrecy to private cubicles where they could enjoy a beauty treatment without fear of publicity.

Towards the end of the century women began to liberate themselves from the mental confines of a restrictive outlook and the woman of personality emerged to replace the demure innocent of the earlier Victorian period. The bevy of attractive and talented actresses who delighted London audiences at this time helped to create this different image of feminine beauty.

Sarah Bernhardt became the idol of the day, encouraging such diverse creative talents as Swinburne and Burne Jones to use her as their inspiration (*Plate 33*). Oscar Wilde likened her profile to that on a Roman coin, and a contemporary critic wrote, 'She has one of those delicate, expressive heads that the illuminators of the Middle Ages painted in the miniatures of their manuscripts. Deep, shining, liquid eyes, a straight fine nose, red lips that open like a flower revealing the sharp whiteness of the teeth, a long flexible neck . . .' (Theodore de Banville.)

Sarah Bernhardt made ample use of cosmetic artifice even outside the theatre. 'While talking to Henry [Irving] she took some red stuff out of her bag and rubbed it on her lips. This frank "making-up" in public was a far more astonishing thing in the 80's than it would be now'. (Ellen Terry.) Bernhardt applied her carmine lip dye with a badger hair brush and from contemporary photographs it is obvious that she used a great deal of white powder and a kohl-like eye make-up.

Ellen Terry's daily use of cosmetics was restricted to darkening her brows and powdering her face—a habit which the impresario Charles Reade tried to break by teasingly referring to her powder puff as 'old chalky'.

The beautiful Jersey actress, Lily Langtry, who also employed artifice, had the distinction of having her fair hair dyed ebony black by the Austrian court hairdresser and his royal master, Crown Prince Rudolf, who was to shock the world a few months later by committing suicide with his mistress at Mayerling. The prince had been an ardent admirer of Lily Langtry, so that when she declared her boredom with her own hair colour, he had responded only too readily. However, the black dye was unreliable and, after the first wash, her own blonde colouring emerged between stripes of vivid heliotrope, and her hair had to be concealed under a wig.

139

Many contemporary women began to turn to the use of artifice as an aid to beauty. Although this may have been in part due to the example set by their favourite actresses, the relaxing of a strict moral climate enabled women to use cosmetics without fear of social censure. Rouged cheeks became more obvious, but lip colouring was still unusual; eyes were enhanced with shadows of kohl made from powdered chalk; lashes were thickened with coconut oil and darkened with 'lamp black' mascara, and nails were lightly coloured with scented red oil and polished with a chamois leather cloth. Home-made beauty preparations were still popular, but an increasing number of purchased cosmetics found their way to the dressing table.

Oscar Wilde comments, in *A Woman of No Importance*, that there were only two kinds of women in society at this time 'the plain and the coloured', and a contemporary undergraduate, Max Beerbohm, writes: 'Nay, but it is useless to protest. Artifice must queen it once more in town. . .' (*In Defence of Cosmetics*, 1896.) Beerbohm welcomes the return of cosmetics as he hopes that an absorption with vanity will replace the growing female interest in masculine sports, such as tennis, golf and cycling, and literary pursuits involving the energetic use of a typewriter. 'With bodily activity their powder will fly, their enamel crack'. However, in spite of his apparent approval of cosmetics, he writes with a certain sad nostalgia: 'For behold! The Victorian era comes to its end and the day of sancta simplicitas is quite ended. The old signs are here and the portents to warn the seer of life that we are ripe for a new epoch of artifice. Are not men rattling the dice-box and ladies dipping their fingers in the rouge-pot?'

CHAPTER NINE

The Twentieth Century
1899-1945

> Beauty, in the old days, used to float into the world like Botticelli's Venus on a shell, natural, breath-taking, divine. Beauty, to-day, is made from baser metals by an astonishing alchemy totally of our time. (*Vogue's Book of Beauty*, 1933)

The new tolerance of cosmetic artifice as an aid to beauty had an increasing effect on the toilet habits of Englishwomen during the final years of Queen Victoria's reign. The era of soap and water, and modest applications of home-made face creams, was certainly at an end.

> 'Make-up' seems to become almost a passion with most women who indulge in it to any extent. There is little room for doubt that the 'art' is largely on the increase. A chemist only the other day remarked to me how much the practice had grown of late. 'Quite young girls come in now,' he said, 'and ask for powder, and even rouge and eyebrow pencils, without the least embarrassment'. (*The Art of Beauty: A Book for Women and Girls*, 1899)

However, in spite of this contemporary evidence, young girls would undoubtedly have only dared to paint their faces in the privacy of the home or at a select gathering of female friends belonging to their own generation. Society might give its approval to the use of powder and rouge by older women, but unmarried girls were expected to rely on the natural attributes of an unpainted complexion. Thus, social mores to a large extent dictated that the ideal of female beauty, later to become fashionable during the Edwardian period, depended on the sophisticated attractions of the mature women who could, without fear of censure, use cosmetic artifice to create the popular image of feminine good looks.

The understated childlike appearance favoured during the early years of Victoria's reign was replaced in the Edwardian era by a preference for the voluptuous, Junoesque beauty of a curvaceous figure, generously bosomed, and a well-rounded face with an almost florid milk and roses complexion. This chocolate-box prettiness was further enhanced by tiny frizzed curls which covered the forehead and by ample tresses of corn-coloured hair piled up under the shadow of an exotic plumed hat.

Women's highly tinted skin tones, which can be seen in the prints and paintings of the day, were largely created by generous applications of rouge contrasting with the chalky whiteness of powder. Most Edwardian society ladies went in for 'enamelling', as making-up was described at the time, and Queen Alexandra set her seal of royal approval on the fashion by painting her face as liberally as any of her contemporaries.

Cecil Beaton allows one a glimpse of the Edwardian woman's cosmetic *toilette* in his book, *The Glass of Fashion*. He describes a childhood visit to his Aunt Jessie, wife of an influential Bolivian minister, whom he finds 'standing in front of a cheval glass, her hair already arranged and the plumes fixed in place, her face a mask of powder and rouge'. The fact that his father apparently disapproved of Aunt Jessie's use of cosmetics rendered them even more 'delightfully shocking' to the small boy, who never ceased to be intrigued by the sight of his favourite aunt with her neck, arms, back and face covered in thick paint—'which by some was called enamel but which my family referred to as whitewash'—her eyelids painted mauve, her cheeks carnation and her lips cerise.

But the unfamiliar practice of making-up was still a mystery to many society ladies and, although they applied powder and rouge to their faces, these embellishments were often amateurish in effect. However, in the new relaxed atmosphere of the Edwardian era, a breed of women emerged in society whose entire livelihood depended on an immaculate appearance. The high-class courtesans, or *demi-mondaines*, soon learnt that the art of making-up was a vitally important part of their way of life. Many of these women were not strictly beautiful, but they made every effort to improve on nature with a clever use of cosmetics applied in an unusual or individual fashion to suit their particular type of face. They dressed expensively, lived in fine houses and were accomplished in the art of conversation and entertainment. They provided a familiar sight at social gatherings, and could be seen in the London parks exercising elegant Borzoi dogs which complemented their own carefully-studied style of appearance.

The courtesan's expertise with powder and paint must have set an example to many well-born ladies of society, whose disapproval of the *demi-mondaine* was no doubt tinged with envy for their apparent mastery over beauty. This skill with make-up was shared by the actresses of the period. This was the age of operetta and music hall entertainment, and the stage produced many attractive, vivacious stars who enhanced their features with artful applications of theatrical paint. Dancer and actress Gabrielle Ray employed face-shaping techniques, shading her features with mushroom-coloured powder and defining her chin with a light dusting of terracotta applied with a hare's foot. Her cheeks were tinted with 'Bois de rose' and coral rouge; the corners of her eyes and nostrils were emphasised with dots of red, green or mauve paint. Gaby Deslys, another star of the day, blanched her face to the colour of a marshmallow and dyed her cheeks magenta. Her lips were carmined and her eyes were shadowed with turquoise powder which was rendered even more startling by the heavy black mascara on her lashes. The exaggerated make-up employed by an actress for her stage appearances was tempered down for daily life and provided other women with an example of how to use cosmetics to achieve a positive effect.

The theatre had a very definite influence on everyday make-up in the early 1900s when Diaghilev's Russian ballet took London by storm. Society was as thrilled with the exciting sets and costumes designed by Leon Bakst as they were with the brilliant choreography and dancing. In particular, the ballet 'Sheherazade' (*Plate 34*) created a sensation which led to such a craze for orientalism that society ladies entertained their guests by posing in 'tableaux vivants' dressed as slave girls. The Eastern influence had an immediate effect on toiletry. Two famous Guerlain perfumes date from this time; 'Shalimar' came on the market in 1916 and 'Mitsouko' in 1919. Both were musky, oriental scents and many other toilet preparations of the day were designed to simulate the exotic properties of Eastern cosmetics. The dramatic stage make-up of the Russian dancers started a craze for coloured or even gilded eye shadows and these were used to match daring evening dresses by French couturier Paul Poiret, who based his designs and vivid colour schemes on Bakst's stage costumes (*Plate 35*). The Diaghilev ballet was to have a lasting influence on cosmetics. From that period to the present day, tinted eye shadows have been on the market and the craze for gilded oriental eye-paint is one which constantly recurs.

The growing respectability of the beauty establishment and the general acceptance of cosmetics made it unnecessary for women of the late Edwardian era to continue manufacturing toilet preparations at home. Whereas in the early years of the century face powders were still being concocted from starch,

4 (*right*) Mme Lubov
Tchernicheva as
'...herazade'. The ballet
started a craze for
...ientalism in the early
1900s and the exotic
stage eye make-up,
illustrated in this
...hotograph, created a
...gue for coloured and
...n gilded eyeshadows.

...*elow left*) Edwardian
...ng dress. Reproduced
...a Harrods fashion
...ogue. The hairstyles
...ated with plumes and
...s show the influence
...shion of Diaghilev's
...rn ballets.

...*elow right*) Elizabeth
...n advertisement of
...920s. The face in
...hotograph ideally
...sents the look of
...eriod. The hair is
...ed short in a smooth
...the eyes are enhanced
...a kohl-like make-up;
...rows plucked, and
...outh painted a
vivid shade.

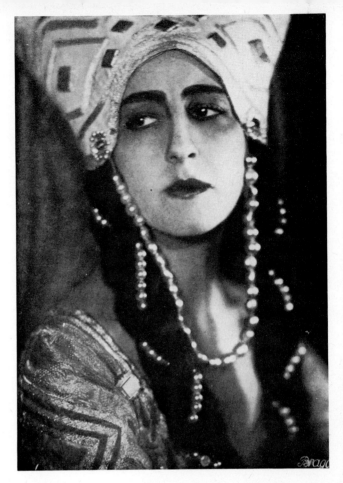

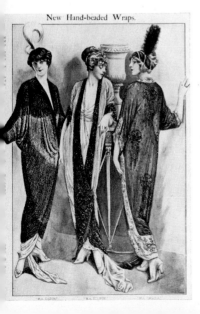

New Hand-beaded Wraps.

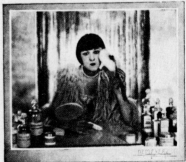

An ELIZABETH ARDEN *Treatment*

Says Elizabeth Arden

THE first step in every treatment of the skin is a thorough
cleansing. This should be done by applying *Venetian
Cleansing Cream* with upward lifting strokes. With just the
warmth of the skin this pure light cream melts into the
pores, where it dissolves and dislodges all the impurities
which clog them, leaving the skin fresh, soft and supple. Then
pat with *Ardena Skin Tonic* to tone, firm and whiten the skin.

VENETIAN CLEANSING CREAM   4 6, 8 6, 12 6
ARDENA SKIN TONIC   3 6, 8 6, 16 6

Write for Elizabeth Arden's book, "*The Quest of the Beautiful*"

ELIZABETH ARDEN

NEW YORK : 673 Fifth Avenue LONDON : 25C, Old Bond Street PARIS : 2, rue de la Paix
Arden Venetian Toilet Preparations are sold at smart shops everywhere

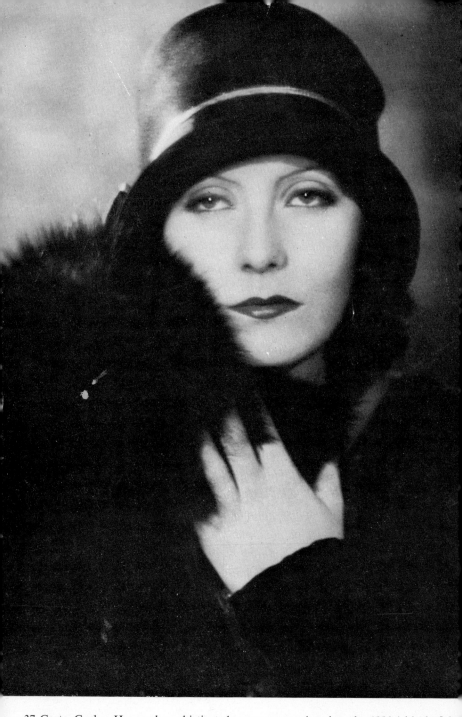

37 Greta Garbo. Her cool, sophisticated appearance epitomises the 1930s' ideal of be
which she helped to create. Pale, unrouged cheeks were fashionable; lipstick shades were
vivid and the line of dark pencil used to emphasise the lid of the eye was Garbo's innova

flour, talc and French chalk, and one beauty book of 1899 even suggested beetroot juice as a rouge for the cheeks, ladies were now determined to rely on the ingenuity of the professional beautician to provide them with a comprehensive range of toiletry. However, although cosmetic manufacturers made every effort to comply with the new demand for a variety of make-up preparations, it was only at a later date that they were totally successful in this respect. Numerous brands of soap and perfume appeared on the market, but cold cream and vanishing cream seem to have been the only concoctions designed for the complexion. Eye shadows, rouge and face powder were produced in only a small range of tints. 'Papier Poudre' in pale pink or mauve was popular, while the white shades and 'Poudre de Riz', made from rice powder, were used as face blanches. Carmine was still the favourite form of rouge.

The new delight in cosmetic artifice focused attention on the head and on the décolletage. The bold bosom then in fashion was frequently emphasised with artificial shadows of powder in the cleavage, whilst delicately etched veins of pale blue paint simulated the perfection of a naturally translucent breast. The purpose of this was to enhance the mature womanliness of the subject; the softly coiled hairstyles gave additional emphasis to femininity.

In the Edwardian period, hair was indeed a woman's crowning glory and, where nature was lacking, artificial padding and false postiches supplemented the deficiency. Blonde or red-gold tresses were once more in vogue and quantities of false locks were imported from Scandinavian and Breton villages, where unfortunate peasant girls were paid a pittance for their hair. Dyes were resorted to by many women who were not naturally fair yet wished to accord with the fashionable ideal of the moment. The effect created by these colouring agents, which were manufactured from henna and cobalt extracts, was anything but subtle or unobtrusive. Even Winston Churchill, when

President of the Board of Trade in 1909, remarked during a society wedding that 'seemingly not one woman in ten can do without hair dye' and he thought the Chancellor of the Exchequer, Lloyd George, should tax this commodity as it would 'yield a vast income'.

The elaborate nature of contemporary hairstyles made a woman dependent on the skill of her maid or on the expertise of a professional hairdresser. Although private visits from the latter were favoured at this time, hairdressing salons were beginning to make an appearance in London. Advances in chemistry had provided these establishments with a range of reliable shampoos, which were a pleasant change from the home-made concoctions of egg used at the turn of the century; but the curling equipment employed on the premises was undeniably primitive.

In 1908, however, M. Marcel from France introduced his famous 'Marcel Wave', which revolutionised hairdressing techniques in England. These were further improved by Karl Nessler's invention of 'permanent waving', then in its infancy but later to become a perfected and reliable form of curling process.

The outbreak of war in 1914 had an immediate effect on women's hairstyles and changed the ideal of feminine beauty. Even before the war, suffragette sympathisers and female intellectuals had attempted to convince their contemporaries that long hair was a symbol of feminine bondage, but it was only when women began to contribute to the war effort by working in factories that, for purely practical reasons, they allowed their hair to be cropped short. Long hair had an unfortunate habit of coming adrift from its pins and combs and falling into factory machinery, which both endangered the life of the individual and halted the production line. As for the luxurious *coiffures* of the leisured age now past, these had no place in wartime England where many women abandoned

146

domestic service to seek work in factories, leaving their former employers with the impossible task of coping with their own long tresses.

World War I accelerated the process of women's emancipation. War work in factories made women realise that the home was not the only place for feminine talents and they now sought positions in commerce and the professions. Class barriers had also, to some extent, disintegrated during the war, as men and women of different social backgrounds worked together for the common good. The new position that women felt they

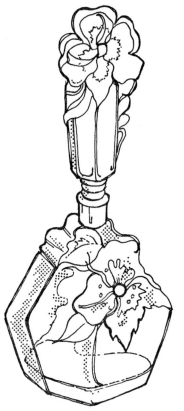

Fig 26 Toilet-water bottle of moulded glass with etched surface and blue-green enamel decoration in the recesses of the design, Lalique, c 1920

147

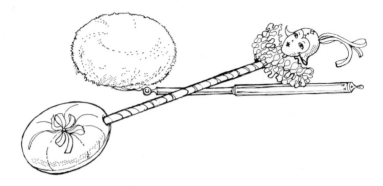

Fig 27 Long-handled powder puffs for powdering the back or face, one of swansdown and satin with chromium-plated telescopic handle, *c* 1930; the other of pink velvet with enamelled porcelain head of a pierrette on pink and black ribbon-covered handle, *c* 1925–30

had acquired in society and the difference in social atmosphere had a profound effect on their looks. Make-up was more widely used than ever before. During the war the working-class girl had come into contact with the cosmetic fashions of the upper classes, and an extensive distribution of reasonably priced toiletry in the shops of post-war England allowed women from every social background to paint their faces according to the fashionable ideals of the day. As a result women's looks became standardised into a classless form of appearance.

Female emancipation, paradoxically, inspired women to make greater use of cosmetics. Although these were applied with a higher degree of art and subtlety, this was quite blatantly done in public. Husbands and menfolk generally were appalled at the sight of their wives and girl friends wielding a powder puff outside the privacy of their own homes but, while women's magazines appealed to their readers to show more appreciation of masculine sensitivity, the habit of making-up in public was here to stay.

Men were to sustain yet another shock to their sensibilities

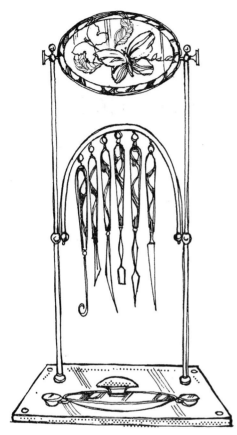

Fig 28 Manicure set on glass base with plated metal stand supporting a bevelled oval mirror, framed in tortoiseshell, and with hooks for suspending the manicure tools, c 1920

with the advent of a new cosmetic fashion. 'A form of make-up which has become deplorably obvious of late is that of rouging the lips. No effort is made to be sparing with the use of the lip-stick. The fashion has come from Paris, of course. It is a pity, because it goes directly against all the canons of successful make-up'. (Rita Strauss, *The Beauty Book*, 1924.) After many years of exile from the world of fashion, vivid lip colouring made its debut in the 1920s and became the most popular form of cosmetic used at the time. The new young generation of

149

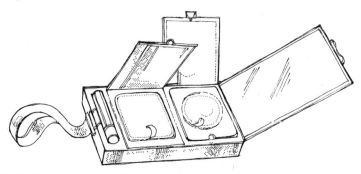

Fig 29 Vanity case in gilt metal with compartments for rouge, powder, comb, lipstick, cigarettes, matches and stamps, Japan, early 1930s

women—the 'flappers' or 'bright young things' of the twenties —used their scarlet lipsticks in a deliberate and, it seems, successful attempt to shock their elders. They were determined in every way to mark themselves out as a generation apart and, even if their originality depended on such trivialities as the use of make-up, this served their purpose. Parental opposition gradually gave way, however, as mothers, determined to keep up with the style of the times, adopted the cosmetic fashions of their daughters.

The new ideal of beauty was dependent on two items of make-up—the lipstick and the eyebrow pencil. Bright artificial colouring was used to paint a 'cupid's bow' shape over the natural form of the mouth, and a thin arched line was pencilled over the eyebrow, which had been either extensively plucked or completely depilated (*Plate 36*). When the cupid's bow became unfashionable, pencilled brows began to get more exaggerated and resembled the winged antennae of some strange insect. Eyebrow pencil was also used to simulate a patch by turning a mole on the face into a painted beauty spot.

The foundation for these cosmetic conceits was still a white complexion emphasised by pale pink powder with a touch of rouge on the cheeks. Eyelids were coloured for evening or glossed with lanolin during the day; lashes were darkened with mascara, and drops of belladonna made from deadly nightshade added a sparkle to the whites of the eye. A framework for the contemporary face was provided by a cropped bob of hair which might well have been dyed to a pale platinum with the aid of one of the latest blonde bleaches.

Essentially, the new style of looks was one which suited a youthful face and figure. The Junoesque form of the Edwardian lady was now out of date; indeed, she would have had a great deal of trouble in squeezing her ample curves into the knee-length, flat-bodiced dresses which were the rage of the moment. It was unfortunate for the older woman that her mature attractions were never again to become truly fashionable. Whereas in the Edwardian era young women had vainly tried to make themselves look older, from the 1920s to the present day women have endeavoured to look permanently young in a world where youth and beauty are thought to be synonymous. The rapid transition from the matronly physique of the Edwardian lady to the slight proportions of the 'flapper' was due, according to some fashion historians, to the heavy loss of men's lives during the war. Young women of the twenties with their youthful faces and boyish figures thus replaced the men who had been killed in battle.

The new desire for a young appearance encouraged cosmetic manufacturers and beauty salons to produce a range of preparations and treatments designed to erase wrinkles, discourage double chins and generally preserve a youthful complexion. Helena Rubinstein, who had established her salon in London in 1908, contributed a number of creams and lotions for this purpose; Cyclax produced a variety of 'Reducing Fluids', 'New Muscle Restorers', forehead straps and chin straps; and Canadian beautician Elizabeth Arden opened her London salon in 1922, introducing Englishwomen to a selection of special creams for different skin types. Her 'Vienna Youth

Masque' treatment was a particular favourite with women during the 1920s. This involved casting plaster replicas of the individual face, after which padded masks were hand-made from the moulds. The masks were electrically wired and the treatment was a form of short-wave therapy which cost sixty guineas.

Face-lifting, as a means of rejuvenation, came into fashion with a vengeance during the twenties and, although plastic surgery was in an elementary stage of development, the experience gleaned from operations on scarred soldiers after the war was to prove an invaluable aid to the advance of cosmetic surgery. Dentists added their expertise to the skill of the plastic surgeon and badly-spaced, stained teeth were corrected or disguised with artificial coverings.

The cosmetic chemist and beautician contributed to the improvement in general standards of appearance by producing make-up of a soft and more subtle consistency. Delicately coloured rouges replaced the cruder dyes of Edwardian England and two popular tints were described in a contemporary beauty book as 'Brunette' and 'Framboise'. Finer blends of powder from natural materials were manufactured for the mass market, but in only three basic shades—pink, natural and 'Rachel'. Endless research was devoted to that most popular cosmetic, the lipstick; new colouring ingredients included carmine dye made from insects found in the Canary Islands and Mexico; Spanish alkanet root, and red lithol salts. The colour was mixed into an oil base of spermaceti, beeswax and lanolin made of fat extracted from the wool of sheep.

The production of better quality cosmetics continued to be the main aim of toiletry manufacturers in the 1930s. By this time the beauty business had become a thriving industry. In 1935 the value of cosmetics produced in England reached the unprecedented figure of £6,769,000 and it was estimated that thirty-five per cent of sales from chemist shops were toiletry preparations. The office girl of 1932 spent what was, in the values of the time, a large part of her weekly salary on cosmetics: 7d on face powder and manicure preparations, 4d on vanishing cream, and 3d each on toilet soap, cleansing lotion, night cream and lipstick (which in 1932 cost 2s and 1s 3d for a refill). Apart from in chemist shops, a comprehensive range of toiletry could be bought in most department stores, and Woolworths had begun to stock a selection of beauty preparations just after World War I.

The ever-growing demand for novel ideas in toiletry encouraged cosmetic manufacturers to introduce an increasing number of new beauty products to the mass market. Elizabeth Arden produced her 'colour harmony' range, an interesting innovation which involved matching make-up to clothes rather than skin tones. In addition, she introduced a more extensive variety of lipstick shades which were later matched up with cream rouges designed to complement the range of lip dyes. The number of tinted face powders on the market also increased. Roger and Gallet produced perfumed powders in shades of white, natural, 'Rachel', 'Rachel Foncée', 'Ocre Rose' and 'Aurore', and even the English chemists, Boots, had extended their modest range of powder to include new colours. Innoxa's comprehensive selection of skin creams included 'Complexion Milk', 'Complexion Vitalizer', 'Skin Tonic' and 'Skin Food'. In 1936 Yardley opened a beauty salon in Bond Street, adding a new variety of toiletry products to their already famous collection of soaps and colognes. 1937 saw the foundation of the cosmetic house of Gala, which at first produced only three lipstick shades, but later captured the younger woman's market by concentrating on the creation of new lip-colours with such dramatic names as 'Lantern Red', 'Blaze' and 'Sea Coral'.

Perfumes at this time were still only considered *chic* if they were imported from France, but these were far too expensive for the ordinary shop girl or office worker. However, in 1936 a man named Douglas Collins provided a solution to the working girl's dilemma. His idea was to manufacture high quality perfumes but reduce their retail price by selling them in small bottles. He began his business at his mother's home in Brighton, marketing his products under the brand name of Goya. Later he obtained four rooms in Whitehorse Street, Piccadilly, but by 1946 the sales of his perfumes warranted the purchase of a factory housed in an eighteenth-century brewery at Amersham in Buckinghamshire. The most famous Goya scents were 'Black Rose' and 'Passport'.

The healthy competition between cosmetic houses and toiletry manufacturers, who were intent on capturing the attention of the mass market, resulted in an enormous increase in advertising. In the second half of 1932 approximately £250,000 was spent on promoting beauty preparations. The largest portion of this expenditure was concentrated on toilet soaps, followed by skin creams, dentifrices, perfumery, face powders and manicure products. Cosmetic houses began to realise that, although advertising was a successful method of encouraging sales of their preparations, attractively designed containers and packaging were equally important. American toiletry manufacturers were ahead of their English equivalents in this respect and had employed the talents of designers like Maurice Levy, who had introduced the first metal containers for cosmetics. However, British beauty firms quickly followed the example of the Americans and made use of the creative skills of artists like Lalique to design their bottles, jars and boxes.

The new large range of attractively packaged cosmetic products must have presented the contemporary woman with a bewildering variety of choice, but magazines and beauty books were quick to provide their readers with hints on which kind of preparation to use for their individual needs or what style of make-up was best suited to their particular type of face. *Vogue*

Beauty Book of 1933 suggested that eyeshadows should match the colour of the eyes although violet or silver tints could be used to provide a touch of glamour for the evening. Blue mascara was considered to be the most flattering, but blue-green was thought to look more natural. False eye lashes, which were now on the market, could be used by the really daring woman, although those of a less adventurous nature might prefer to curl their natural lashes with the aid of 'a little eyelash iron'. *Vogue*'s advice to its readers concentrated on the importance of a youthful figure, which could be acquired with the help of electrical massage now available at many beauty salons, and articles entitled 'The Skin Game' insisted that 'no beauty can be a beauty today without a good skin'.

A pale complexion had become fashionable once more. Magazines insisted that the bright pink cheeks of the pre-war era were totally out of date. The new ideal in feminine looks was vaguely reminiscent of the Middle Ages and depended on good facial bone structure, thinly arched brows and a pure white skin. *Vogue* stated that 'some of to-day's beauties haven't any more natural colour in their faces than a handkerchief' and although a light blush of rouge could be used in moderation, lipstick provided the main colour emphasis to the face.

Contemporary men may well have approved of this new type of pale femininity. Thus, in Noël Coward's *Private Lives*, when Amanda informs Victor that she intends to acquire a Riviera sun tan, he is immediately unenthusiastic:

> *Victor:* 'I hate sunburnt women.'
> *Amanda:* 'Why?'
> *Victor:* 'It's somehow, well, unsuitable.'
> *Amanda:* 'It's awfully suitable to me, darling.'

However, unfortunately for Amanda, sunburnt complexions were not to become fashionable till a later date as a healthy suntan would have been at a variance with the whole look of the

1930s, which was one of cool, urbane sophistication, more adult than the twenties and dependent on elegant, immaculate grooming.

The cinema began to have a positive influence on feminine looks and one film star in particular possessed a type of beauty which was so carefully copied that, to a large extent, it created the style of appearance typical of the thirties. Greta Garbo's pale enigmatical features and her highly individual approach to make-up were admired by female audiences all over England (*Plate 37*). Cecil Beaton states that 'Before Garbo, faces were pink and white. But her very simple and sparing use of cosmetics completely altered the face of the fashionable woman'. (*The Glass of Fashion*.) One innovation which Garbo introduced was the accentuation of the upper eyelid with a line of black eyebrow pencil and many women began to use this cosmetic effect in lieu of tinted eye shadow.

Other film stars like Norma Shearer, Jean Harlow and Madeleine Carroll also had an influence on contemporary ideals of beauty. Thus there began to be a demand for toilet preparations which enabled the girl in the street to emulate the glamorous appearance of a Hollywood star. Cosmetic toothpastes, which emphasised the whiteness of the teeth by tinting the gums pink, appeared on the market, so that any woman could now charm her husband or boy friend with one of those dazzling smiles she had observed on the screen. But a flash of white teeth was not enough, in her view, to create the perfect image. She coveted the brightly-coloured gleaming lipsticks which her favourite stars used in their film roles. These were provided for the Englishwoman's use by Hollywood cosmetician, Max Factor, who opened his first beauty salon in London in 1936. Using his vast experience of film make-up as a guide, he introduced a large variety of lipstick and powder shades to the mass market. Lipsticks with a shiny finish became all the rage and many other toiletry manufacturers, like the French firm of Lancôme, produced successful versions of this type of cosmetic.

The film world popularised yet another cosmetic innovation —nail varnish. The vogue for painting fingernails had originated in Paris society and amongst the French èlite who haunted Riviera resorts in the summer, but it only came to the notice of the general female public when film stars began to adopt the fashion. The idea was immediately popular and, although some women restricted themselves to the use of pale pink polish, the more adventurous used brighter colours. 'Cardinal', 'Garnet' and 'Coral' were favourite shades of varnish, but some American women were audacious enough to paint their fingernails black. In England, the deep vivid shades of red only became generally accepted in 1936, and by 1938 toenails were also being painted to draw attention to the open-toed evening sandals which were then fashionable. At this date the colour range of varnishes increased to seven shades, but *Vogue* was insistent that 'the blood shades are brilliant and decorative in the evening but a little too, too violent for the light of day'.

Magazines, advertisements and films promoted an image of beauty which made women increasingly aware of their looks and any shortcomings they might have in comparison. As a result they spent more time in beauty salons and hairdressers to ensure that they were perfectly groomed. At home, their dressing tables were covered in pots and jars, scents in cut-glass spray bottles and face powder in ornate glass bowls. Eyebrow pencils, mascara brushes, lipsticks and eyeshadows shared space with containers of depilatory wax and cream or liquid deodorants.

Women's self-conscious attitude to beauty made them aware of the appearance of their masculine escorts and articles on 'Improving Your Husband' were popular reading at the time. The Englishman might well have appeared immaculate in his own eyes: tastefully dressed in his London club or in manly

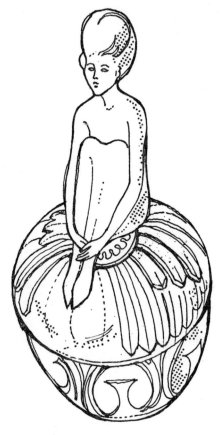

Fig 30 Powder bowl press-moulded in pale green glass and acid etched to achieve a frosted effect, with lid in the form of a bathing girl sitting on two shells, *c* 1930

tweeds on the golf course, with sensibly cut, short hair. His wife, however, was determined to improve his standard of grooming and was encouraged in this by magazines which suggested he should use Continental perfumes instead of his lightly scented after-shave lotions. They also insisted that a husband secretly made use of his wife's face powder, so why should he not be provided with the 'after-shave powder' which was now on the market. There was also an 'after-shave cream' which his wife could persuade him to use by insisting that it was an excellent way of soothing a chapped skin after a windy day on the golf course. The Englishman, however, defeated both his wife and the magazine journalists by maintaining a spartan attitude to his *toilette*.

The Englishwoman's delight in vanity suffered a severe blow with the outbreak of war in 1939. Cosmetic houses in America continued to supply their female customers with beauty preparations to boost morale during the war, but the English girl often had to rely on a stiff and unpainted upper lip as cosmetics became increasingly hard to obtain. The 'Limitations of Supplies Order' of 1940 cut down cosmetic materials to a minimum because the petroleum and alcohol necessary for the manufacture of toiletry was required for war purposes. Thus fewer beauty preparations could be manufactured and the factories' change-over to war work further restricted their production. Yardley's factory was used for manufacturing aircraft components and sea water purifiers, whilst Cyclax employed their expertise to invent a special sunproof cream which was supplied to the War Office for soldiers fighting in hot climates. They also provided a cosmetic paint which was mixed with green stain and used by the army as a camouflage dye. This same cosmetic paint formed the basis for 'Cyclax Stockingless Cream', a preparation designed to replace the sheer stockings that were now rationed. Englishwomen coloured their legs with the dye, after which a 'seam' was drawn down the back of each 'stocking' with a black eyebrow pencil—a service no doubt performed by a helpful girlfriend to ensure that the line was straight.

The extraordinary adaptability of the English in a time of crisis was admirably illustrated by the list of cosmetic substitutes supplied to girls in His Majesty's Forces. It was appreciated that make-up was essential to feminine morale, and although generally frowned on in the women's services, cosmetics could be worn 'with discretion'. A bizarre selection of skin cleansers and colouring agents were suggested in lieu of conventional beauty preparations. Lemon juice, methylated spirit, potato flesh, the water from fruit parings, egg-white were encouraged for toning the complexion and egg-yolk as a shampoo, while vegetable oil was recommended as a foundation for face powder. Even women who were not in the forces had to improvise with home-made cosmetics, as lipsticks were often only obtainable on the black market and such necessary articles as toilet soaps were rationed.

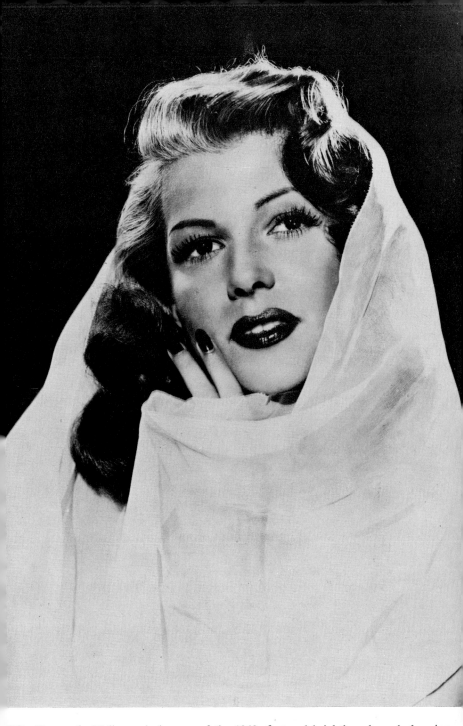

Rita Hayworth. Hollywood glamour of the 1940s featured brightly coloured gleaming and long varnished nails, which were copied by women everywhere.

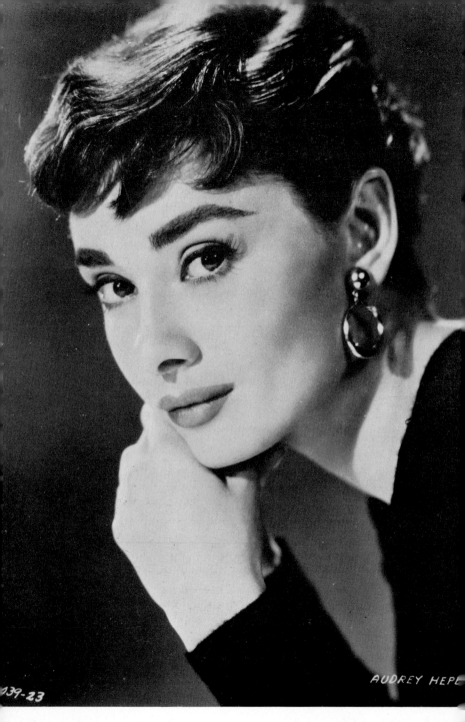

AUDREY HEPL

139-23

39 Audrey Hepburn. Her whimsical, gamin type of beauty set the fashion in the late 195
She emphasised her eyes with an exaggerated use of black eyeliner and accentuated her e
brows with dark pencil. To focus attention on her eyes, she used a very pale lipstick.

CHAPTER TEN

The Twentieth Century
1945-1970s

Today's very latest name of the game in eye make-up. From Elizabeth Arden. The most spectacular spread of mood-matching colours you've ever gazed on. Twenty-four tantalizing shades. All the way from pretty cool to out-and-out wild. And such textures . . . clear and creamy for Powder cream Shadows. Shimmer and sparkle, the Powder frosts. The Ultra frosts, all dazzle and zing. Your own eye make-up extravaganza. To dabble in. To do your own eye-thing with. Beautifully. (Advertising copy for Elizabeth Arden's 'Self Portrait Eyes' 1972)

After the war and with the end of rationing, the commercial world of fashion and beauty created a new image of femininity for contemporary women. The military uniforms of girls in the forces and the utility dress of wartime England had camouflaged the softer aspects of a feminine appearance. With the possible exception of hairstyles like the romantic 'page boy' bob inspired by film star Veronica Lake, women had looked like poor copies of their masculine counterparts. The unavailability of toiletry and cosmetics had contributed to this spartan image. Thus, when wartime restrictions ended, women longed for the return of essentially feminine fashions in dress and cosmetics.

Responding to this demand, Paris couturier Christian Dior introduced his 'New Look' in 1947. It was in every way the antithesis of wartime utility dress. The shoulder line was softer, waists were nipped in, and skirts were long and voluminous involving a lavish use of fabric which would have been impossible during the war. Beauty houses correspondingly produced a wide range of 'New Look' cosmetics to complement this fashion and the variety of toiletry products now available was greater than before the war.

A study of cosmetic advertisements in 1948 and 1949 gives some indication of the diversity of beauty preparations manufactured at this time. The main emphasis was on colour and novelty packaging. Elizabeth Arden produced a large variety of matching lipstick and nail polish colours. Rimmel introduced an ingenious palette of lip colour which incorporated a mirror and brush. Goya, venturing into the field of cosmetics, produced their 'Thick and Thin' lipstick. This consisted of two metal lipstick containers, one slim and one thick, joined together by a delicate chain. The narrow lip-pencil was used to outline the lips while the other filled them in with a generous application of colour. Gala introduced a lipstick innovation to the mass market in their 'lipline' pencil. The container for this product, like the Goya lipstick, was its main selling feature. It was designed to enable women to apply their lip colour with a new degree of control and in the words of an enthusiastic journalist: 'The very newest lipstick is not a lipstick, but a real lip pencil—long and slender, and sheathed in a bright gold case. No more smudges as long as you can keep a fairly steady hand. And you should get a clearer, better line, because it really is easier to use.' (*Glasgow Citizen*, 1948). The 'lipline' pencil was manufactured in Gala's new range of colours, which included the old favourites 'Blaze' and 'Lantern Red', with matching nail polishes in 'non-spill' bottles.

The majority of beauty advertisements at this time concentrated on lipsticks or nail varnishes. These were obviously the most popular cosmetics as they were essential to the new style of appearance. The fashionable ideal of femininity in the late 1940s was one of brittle elegance and superficial glamour— an image of beauty borrowed from the film world. Max Factor was using film stars for his advertisements and top French models were also employed to promote cosmetics. Their scarlet lips and long, gleaming nails were considered *chic* and even feminine (*Plate 38*).

The new appearance to which women aspired was in part due to the influence of films but owed a great deal to the emancipated role of women in society. Ever since World War I, the old-fashioned idea of femininity had gradually changed. In the thirties women had begun to see themselves as cool sophisticates influenced by the detached, enigmatic approach to life of film stars like Greta Garbo. By 1940 more women had substituted office for home giving them the detachment of financial independence. The film star image had exerted an even greater influence on their imagination. Thus woman's ideal had altered from the submissive role of the Victorian housewife to the role of a glamorous, worldly seductress.

The whole image of 'glamour', which largely depended on a superficial and artificially produced type of beauty, created an unprecedented demand for toilet preparations. It is undoubtedly true, for instance, that the blonde goddesses of the screen, who introduced the idea of sex appeal to the public, inspired women to buy a much greater quantity of peroxide bleaches. Women had become more capricious in their tastes and were no longer content to devote their loyalty to one type of make-up or skin cream. So beauty houses began to market an ever-changing variety of cosmetics. During the war Englishwomen had 'made do' with a limited number of toiletry products. Now they demanded not only variety but good quality and effective results from their skin creams and lotions. They quickly discovered that certain beauty houses produced particularly suitable preparations for English complexions. Thus, Elizabeth

Arden, Yardley and Ponds enjoyed an especially good reputation at this time. Styles of make-up also began to change more rapidly than they had in the past. As a result the popular ideal in feminine looks was modified with each new type of cosmetic fashion. There was no longer a standardised image of beauty which lasted for any length of time.

Although new lipstick and eyeshadow colours constantly appeared in the shops, powder was still basically designed to create a pink and white complexion. However, in the late 1950s Gala produced a new shade of powder and foundation which was based on yellow and pink colouring ingredients. The result was a beige face make-up which Gala cleverly christened 'Mutation Mink'. The name was designed to evoke thoughts of a Rolls-Royce and diamond tiaras—a snob appeal that immediately captured the imagination of the mass market. This make-up was best suited to darker skinned women, but it toned down the pinkest 'English rose' complexion to the deeper shades of a Continental skin. Other cosmetic houses were producing a selection of dark or more subtly tinted powders and foundations, and these created a new diversity of artificial complexion colours.

One reason for this innovation in powder shades was the realisation that each individual type of complexion was attractive in its own right. A pink or white make-up might suit the true 'English rose' colouring, but it only camouflaged the often distinctive beauty of a dark or even sallow skin. The new variety of powders and foundations enabled each woman to enhance her own special kind of looks.

There was another more interesting reason for this new make-up—the contemporary fashion for a darker complexion. For centuries a white skin had remained a desirable feature of beauty. Judging from the poetry, drama and prose of the past it was considered the most important physical attribute that any woman could possess. A brown skin was a characteristic

164

of the country peasant who had to work in the fields for a living. Therefore a suntan was a sign of humble social origins whereas a carefully tended pale complexion was an indication of a leisured aristocratic life. However, by the twentieth century, society had changed and it had also became fashionable to travel abroad to coastal resorts in the summer. People began to enjoy a new pastime—sunbathing. A bronzed complexion was now considered attractive not only for its own sake but because it indicated that the individual had just spent an expensive holiday on the Continent—an advantage which, before the days of the package tour, was not available to 'Everyman'. Thus, a suntanned skin was considered *chic*—an enviable characteristic of the Riviera élite. Sun oils and creams became increasingly popular. These were designed to protect the skin from over-exposure to the sun's rays and allowed women to tan their skins safely without burning themselves to the colour of a well-boiled lobster. It is amusing to reflect that in French or Italian peasant communities, even today, women still believe in the long out-moded idea that a white skin betokens gentle birth and is more beautiful than a skin which has been exposed to the sun. Unlike the modern tourist who makes strenuous efforts to acquire a bronzed tan, the French peasant woman, whenever possible, shades her complexion from the sun.

During the 1950s, the range of face powders and foundations was matched by an equal variety of lipstick, eyeshadow and nail varnish colours. The dark, vivid red lip-colourings of the 1940s were replaced by paler tints, which may well have been designed to enhance the beauty of a summer suntan by contrasting with the darker tone of the skin. Also, if used in conjunction with one of the deeper shaded or beige face powders, they could simulate a summer complexion even during the winter months. A popular selection of pale colours was produced by Gala who, following the example of Continental cosmeticians, added titanium to their lipsticks to give them a white gleaming appearance on application. 'Italian Pink' was a great favourite from this range. They also manufactured a large number of middle tone colours and one of these was their best-selling lipstick 'Sari Peach'. When it came on the market in the fifties, a joint promotion was organised with *Vogue* who, in one issue of the magazine, selected the colours of clothes to co-ordinate with this new lipstick shade—a type of promotional idea subsequently repeated on many other occasions. Paler lipsticks were also produced by other cosmetic houses. A comprehensive range was available at low prices from Woolworths, while Orlane, Dior and Lancôme catered for more expensive tastes.

Softer coloured lip shades made the mouth a less noticeable feature of the face than during the days of scarlet lipstick. Therefore more attention was focused on the eyes. The enormous range of eyeshadow colours now available were sold in cream or compressed powder form and some were even designed like a child's paintbox to be applied with water and brush. Others resembled coloured crayons contained in metal holders. Glitter eye shadows, whose sparkling effect was made by adding fish scales to the colouring ingredients, were extremely popular.

The most important change in eye make-up was effected by the exaggerated use of black line to emphasise the upper lid of the eye. The old-fashioned eyebrow pencil had been super-seded by an innovation aptly described as 'eye liner'. This was a liquid form of cosmetic paint which was contained in a small bottle and was applied with a brush. It was neater and in many ways easier to use than eyebrow pencil. Women became really adventurous with this make-up, employing it to accentuate the lid and elongate the corners of the eye, which as a result became the most made-up and dominant feature of the con-temporary face. The studied application of this make-up bore more resemblance to the eye decoration of ancient Egypt than anything in English cosmetic history.

This extreme cosmetic fashion had, once again, been due to the influence of a film star. Audrey Hepburn's whimsical and gamine type of beauty captivated film audiences of the day. Her cropped 'urchin' hair-cut drew attention to her delicate features and to her large dark eyes, which were outlined in black paint so that they resembled those of an exotic gazelle, while her natural brows were accentuated with dark pencil (*Plate 39*).

Audrey Hepburn initiated the fashion for a style of appearance which owed more to the Parisian left bank than to the American Hollywood image of feminine glamour. English girls were particularly attracted by the Continental type of beauty seen in European films and attempted to acquire this 'international' look through their own use of cosmetics. In the early 1960s heavy black eye make-up combined with the use of, in many cases, white lipstick, contrived to turn the English girl into a 'pale and interesting' French existentialist student. A bizarre touch was added by contemporary nail varnish colours, especially designed for the young market, which ranged from yellow, green, blue and lilac to jet black.

Youth was to have a much greater influence on cosmetic fashions during the sixties. The advent of 'rock 'n' roll' from America led to a new kind of popular music created for and by the young. The teenage population made it an essential part of their youth cult and in time a whole new style of dress, hairstyles and cosmetics was designed for youthful tastes. The most significant change in appearance was in the length of men's hair. The 'short back and sides' was replaced by a more luxuriant growth of locks. The older generation was at first appalled by these, as they believed, effeminate fashions. It is to be noted, however, that throughout the entire history of English fashion there were basically only two periods when men had short hair—the Middle Ages and the twentieth century. In both cases this was a result of military campaigns. The crusader knight had his hair cut to suit the climate of the Holy Land, and during the two World Wars Englishmen were subjected to army regulation hair cuts which continued to be fashionable in peace time. Perhaps this reversion to what historically has been a normal feature of the Englishman's appearance is a more accurate explanation for men's wish to grow their hair long than, as some sociologists would have it, the preponderance of young males over females—so prompting the need to attract feminine attention—or the revolt of one generation against the conventions of its parents. At the same time, an increase of interest in men's toiletry and the greater care devoted to appearance once more reverted to an older tradition.

The need to capture the attention of the frequently capricious young market constantly taxed the ingenuity of toiletry manufacturers during the sixties. Apart from the teenage demand for make-up, the busy young career girl also required a range of cosmetics which were quick and easy to use. Beauty houses began to concentrate on products which were neatly packaged, expedient to apply and small enough to carry in a handbag for use during the day. Helena Rubinstein's 'mascara-matic', which dispensed with the old-fashioned block mascara applied by brush and water, was immediately popular. It was about the size of a fountain pen. A semi liquid mixture of mascara and preservatives was contained in one end of the 'pen'. The other end held a narrow applicator resembling a slim wand intertwined with a coil of metal. The mascara fixed to the wand and was then applied to the lashes. The 'mascara-matic' was the forerunner of many other types of brushless mascaras, although modern versions contradict this description by substituting a narrow circular brush for the metal applicator. 'Instant' face make-up was much in demand and, although the all-in-one powder and foundation, contained in a simple compact, had been designed at an earlier date, it was particularly favoured at this time.

Cosmetics which created an instant effect and dispensed with old-established beauty routines became increasingly popular. Wearing false nails allowed women to escape from the conventional manicure which had required patience and attention. The application of false eyelashes provided a convenient if artificial alternative to the laborious process of curling natural lashes with old-fashioned devices. New types of home beauty preparations enabled women to avoid, if they wished, spending time in a professional salon. These products, unlike the 'home-made' cosmetics of the past, were mass-produced in factories but designed to be used at home. A wide selection of face mask treatments were now available made from simple natural ingredients like lemon, oatmeal and lanolin. The perfected design of contemporary hair dyes, semi-permanent colours and tinting shampoos, produced by Focus, Inecto and Elida, made it possible for women to colour their own hair yet achieve a professional result. Shampoos were created and classified as suitable for normal, oily or dry hair. Hair lacquer, conditioning creams and medicated treatments were produced so that women could keep their hair in a manageable state without having to depend entirely on the services of a hairdressing salon.

Few women could dispense with the skills of a professional hairdresser when it came to cutting the hair. English salons had benefited from learning Continental cutting and styling techniques and were now able to add innovations of their own. Fashions in hairstyles changed rapidly during the 1960s. Women discovered that fashion had outstripped them and their hair was short when it needed to be long. False postiches, wigs and half-wigs were used to simulate the right length of hair and these could be quickly rejected should short cropped locks return to popularity. The almost unanimous response by women to the caprices of fashion produced a degree of uniformity in hairstyles in the 1960s. Perhaps this was because all women wished to have the same fashionable style when it became the vogue. Or perhaps hairdressers imposed their latest coiffure on too many women at the same time. Whatever the reason, the London streets were filled with women, their skilfully-cut hair cropped into elaborate topiary-like shapes, who looked very similar in appearance.

A desire to conform to an accepted ideal of beauty also encouraged many contemporary women to have their faces altered with cosmetic surgery. A turned up nose could now be straightened, protruding ears flattened and skin skilfully lifted to erase any hint of wrinkling. In short, a modern plastic surgeon could disguise age or rebuild a face to suit the mood of the individual.

Cosmetic manufacturers added their expertise to the specialised talents of the cosmetic surgeon and produced face lotions, moisturisers, nourishing creams and stimulants that catered for every age group or skin type. Their composition, based on the results of painstaking chemical research, contained every possible kind of natural and synthetic ingredient. A hormone cream manufactured by Organon Laboratories had come on the market and sold under the brand name of 'Endocil'. This was considered to be especially suitable for older women, whose natural hormone activity is on the decline. The varied price range of complexion creams enabled women of every income group to afford a good skin preparation. Helena Rubinstein, Elizabeth Arden and Lancôme catered for the higher income brackets; Yardley for the middle income group, and Boots for the moderately-salaried office girl.

The unprecedented variety of cosmetic preparations on the market resulted in an extraordinary diversity of beauty advertisements. Selling their products was an understandable obsession with beauty houses. Advertising agencies, market research experts and public relations consultants were employed to help in the promotion of new cosmetic ideas (*Plate 40*).

Attractive packaging in aerosol containers, plastic tubes or neatly designed cosmetic jars was an essential part of any promotional campaign. Clever advertising copy and exciting visual presentation could make all the difference between the

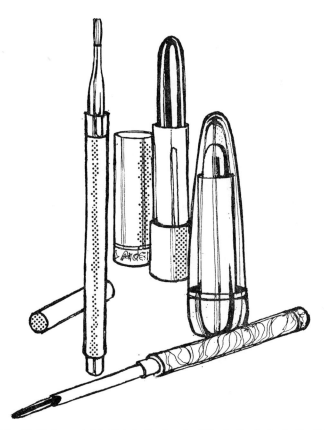

Fig 31 (*left to right*) Coty's lip brush, Elizabeth Arden's lipstick, Yardley's lipstick, and Gala's 'lip pen', a 1970s' version of the earlier Gala 'lipline'

171

success or failure of a product. However, one of the most important selling features of a toiletry commodity is its individual product name. This can conjure up an image or create an association of ideas in the minds of the buying public. An evocative name can enhance a scent with the quality of either romance or nostalgia and endow the most commonplace cosmetic with an aura of mystique borrowed from some historical period associated with a legend of beauty. Snob appeal, sexual adventure and oriental mystery can be evoked by the imaginative choice of one word or a simple title, whose inherent promise of social success or Eastern enchantment is the most effective method of selling the product.

Perfumes frequently have the most evocative names. 'Je Reviens' hints at the nostalgia of a lover's reunion; 'L'Air du Temps' at the sylvan beauty of a summer wood, and 'L'Aimant' the promise of romance. 'Bal à Versailles' recalls the splendour of the French court and 'Le Coq d'Or' is yet another reminder, by Guerlain, of the exotic Eastern ballet introduced by Diaghilev. Scents with the simplest names very often have the most snob appeal, but this depends on the originator of the perfume. Thus, Chanel could afford to label her famous scent, 'No. 5', while the plain initial 'Y' refers to a scent created by Paris couturier, Yves St Laurent. In men's toiletry the same rule applies; 'Arden for Men' or 'A Gentleman's Cologne' seem spartan in their simplicity, but the image they create is instantly expensive and exclusive. Masculine animal virility is implied by names like 'Brut' or 'Cougar', whilst 'Old Spice' has a more comfortable, homely image. Women's lipsticks manufactured for the expensive market are often distinguished by numbers or a simple shade reference, whereas cheaper lipsticks have names which are a great deal more 'expensive' than the selling price.

In the early 1970s the names of complexion creams and make-up indicate a preference for clinical simplicity. A hint of

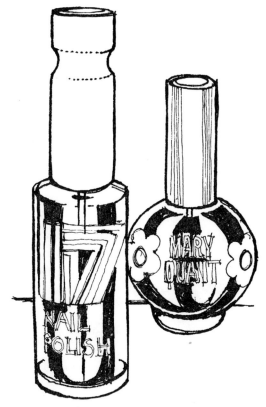

Fig 32 Bottles of nail varnish (*left*) Boots Number
17 (*right*) from Mary Quant

medically-analysed ingredients, vitamin-packed goodness or
herbal purity is much more likely to guarantee sales than any
hint of Eastern promise. In fact, the romantic names given to
cosmetics in the past would be totally unacceptable to the
modern market. A direct hard selling approach which unites
sexual success with beauty has proved popular, but many manufacturers have discovered that emphasis on the 'medicinal'

aspect produces an even greater response in women. Skin treatments with names like 'Natural Organic Skin Care' (Ultima 11); 'Skin Life Biological Anti-Wrinkle Treatment' (Helena Rubinstein), and 'Swedish Formula Hypo-Allergenic Treatment Collection' (Max Factor) might sound like cosmeticians' tongue-twisters but are apparently memorised by the beauty-conscious modern woman. Allergy-tested cosmetics, like the Almay and Clinique range, though specially designed for women with skin allergy problems, are used more generally.

Make-up is named with a contrived plainness, a deliberate attempt, in a feminist age, to shed its ultra-feminine glamour image of the early twentieth century. 'Starkers', a face make-up by Mary Quant; 'Blush-on', a rouge by Revlon, and a host of preparations simply described as 'glosses', 'shiners' or 'blushers' have replaced those earlier exotically titled cosmetics.

The modern face has benefited from the example of film

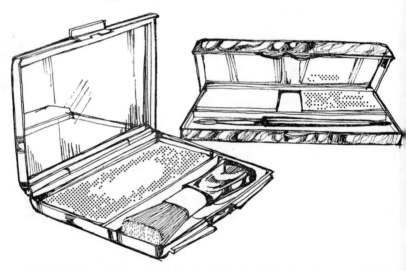

Fig 33 Modern make-up palettes (*left*) Revlon's 'Blush on' rouge, (*right*) Elizabeth Arden's 'Self-Portrait Eyes'

174

and television make-up techniques. These ideas have been translated into the everyday application of cosmetics. Manufacturers have produced a whole series of make-ups and cosmetic tools which enable a woman to bring out the individual character of her face. Eyeshadows, rouges and face preparations, compactly packaged in neat palettes and boxes, come in a variety of colours and textures, and a wide selection of ingeniously designed brushes are provided for use with these make-ups. Beauty writers are constantly advising women on how to emphasise bone structure with artificial shadowing or how to bring out the shape and colour of their eyes by means of light or dark, shiny or matt eyeshadows. The subtle consistency of modern make-up and the wide range of unusual colour combinations allow modern women to employ these 'face-shaping' techniques with artful originality.

It is interesting to appreciate how the modern cosmetic manufacturer, now part of a massive and complex industry, copes with a high volume of output yet maintains a consistent standard of product quality. Sophisticated and efficient factory machinery has helped to produce the required volume of cosmetic preparations, but chemical research, attention to hygiene, and specialised skills are needed to maintain a uniform level of quality.

Yardley's, at Basildon in Essex, is a good example of a modern cosmetic factory. Specialised machines produce two hundredweight of face powder or half a ton of compressed powder and foundation at a time. Vast metal blenders, resembling giant food mixers, can in one mixing vat stir up enough basic colouring substance to manufacture 40,000 lipsticks, and 20,000 individual lipsticks are produced daily. In spite of the enormous volume of production, each quantity of powder, face cream or lipstick is painstakingly examined for bacterial contamination and to ensure that the colour or texture is up to standard. A top dermatologist is often

175

consulted on the composition of new cosmetic compounds to make sure that these are unlikely to cause any skin allergies.

Fresh consignments of lipstick, whose shades are already on the market, are colour matched with the prototypes, manufactured to an exact standardised formula and produced by a meticulous process. The coloured molten wax is poured into a series of tiny moulds contained in a metal casing. These 'embryo' lipsticks are then subjected to a rigorous system of temperature tests. They emerge from their moulds as a finished product except for the process of 'flaming'. This involves sending the lipsticks down a narrow conveyor belt to roll through tiny flames at a great speed. Thus, an outer coat of the wax mixture melts and then dries again to a gleaming finish. Each lipstick has now acquired a shining, polished coating.

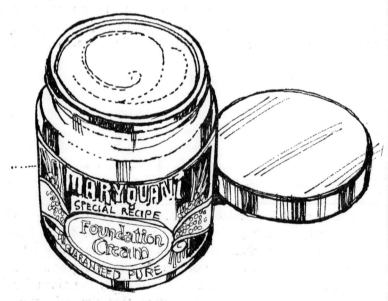

Fig 34 Mary Quant's 'Special Recipe' foundation cream in a glass jar with bright yellow plastic lid

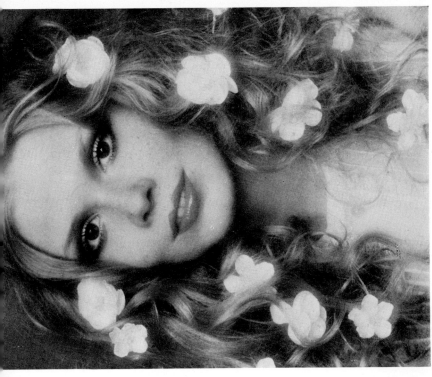

advertisement heralded a new approach to cosmetic advertising in the 1960s.

41 (*right*) Boots face make-up advertisement from 'The Seven Faces of Number Seven' series. A carefully contrived make-up gives the impression of natural looks.

A
WOMAN'S
AMMUNITION...
Go great guns with Yardley lipstick
Be dashing...be exciting,
be captivating. Be fore-armed for
every possible occasion.
And then you can set your sights
as high as you like.
Choose from these sixteen
sure-fire lipsticks.

YARDLEY LIPSTICKS

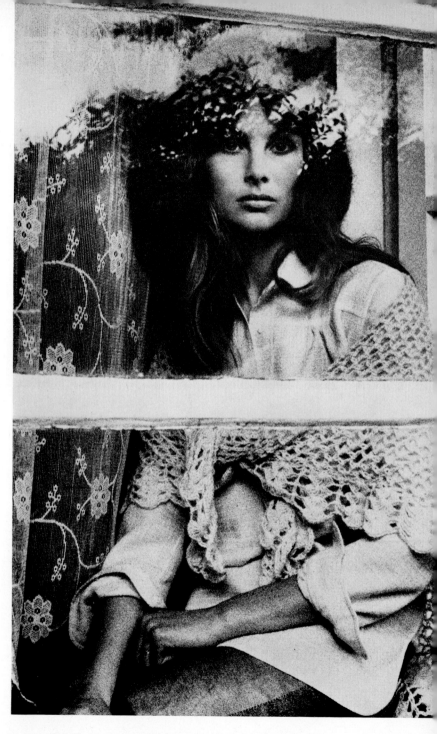

42 Jean Shrimpton photographed at the window of her country cottage. A classic ex
of the modern natural ideal of beauty.

Although the manufacturing methods employed in a modern cosmetic factory would have astounded an ancient Egyptian or Elizabethan, many of the ingredients used in modern beauty products would have appeared familiar to them. Talc and rice powder still form the basis of face powders. Natural waxes, oils and fats are employed as binding agents in the manufacture of all-in-one face make-ups and eyeshadows, and as the main

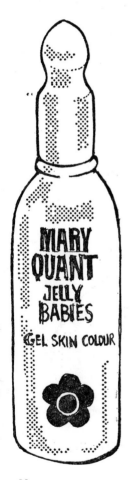

Fig 35 White plastic bottle for Mary Quant's 'Jelly Babies' skin colour

compounds in lipstick and complexion creams. Colouring ingredients are manufactured from basic earth pigments, iron oxides, charcoals and various ochres. The familiar red ochre, which has been used from the beginnings of civilised antiquity as a cosmetic colouring, is still employed for the same purpose today. However, synthetic materials are also used in modern cosmetics. The 'pearlised' lipstick is no longer manufactured from fish scales, but from an artificially produced silver substance whose glinting microscopic facets reflect the light and give the lips a shining effect.

It is interesting that, in a scientific age, natural cosmetic ingredients have not been completely replaced by synthetic substitutes. In part, this is due to the undoubted efficiency of natural materials which thus require no replacement. But, as in the past, even make-up is affected by the influences of contemporary ideals and fashions. The modern fetish for health food and the desire to preserve the natural environment from technological change have turned 'synthetic' into a derogatory word. The 'natural' cosmetic made from herbs and vegetable

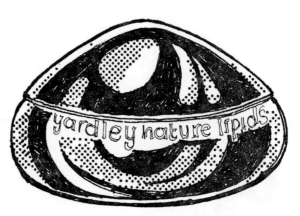

Fig 36 Black plastic container for Yardley's 'Lipid' moisturiser cream

substances, and scented with the natural perfume of thyme, rosemary and marjoram or pine woods and fruit, is more acceptable to modern tastes. Beauty preparations contained in jars which would be more at home in a country larder; cosmetic names, like 'Jelly Babies' by Mary Quant, which are nostalgic reminders of a country sweet shop, and creams like Yardley's natural 'Lipids', designed to reproduce the skin's own moisturising process, are the distinctive products of make-up manufactured in the early 1970s.

Thus modern cosmetics often purport to create a 'natural' look, employing bronze jellies to give an instant healthy, tanned appearance to the skin; eyeshadows and lipsticks which owe their inspiration to the colours of cottage garden flowers and wild berries; and rouges and face make-ups which emulate the glow of a windswept complexion (*Plates 41, 42*). But these clever simulations of natural beauty are far removed from the appearance of a truly 'natural' face, which would be totally devoid of cosmetics. Human vanity, stimulated by the dictates of fashion, perennially ensures that even when ideals of beauty turn to nature for inspiration, her true aspect is masked by the artificial face.

Bibliography

GENERAL SOURCES

Ellis, Aytoun. *The Essence of Beauty* (1960)
Garland, Madge. *The Changing Face of Beauty* (1957)
Gombrich, E. H. J. *The Story of Art* (1966)
Laver, James. *Costume* (1963)
—— *Dandies* (1968)
—— *Modesty in Dress* (1969)
Piper, David T. *The English Face* (1957)
Poucher, William A. *Perfumes, Cosmetics and Soaps* (1959)
Williams, Neville James. *Powder and Paint* (1957)
Woodforde, John. *The Strange Story of False Hair* (1971)
Wright, Lawrence. *Clean and Decent* (1957)
Yarwood, Doreen. *Outline of English Costume* (1970)

CHAPTER ONE THE ORIGINS OF COSMETICS

Bradley, Carolyn. *A History of World Costume* (1964)
Elkin, A. P. *The Australian Aborigines* (Angus & Robertson, Sydney, 1966)
Faris, James C. *Nuba Personal Art* (1972)
Hiler, Hilaire. *From Nudity to Raiment* (1929)
Josephy, A. M. *The American Heritage Book of Indians* (1968)
Strathern, Andrew and Marilyn. *Self-Decoration in Mount Hagen* (1971)

CHAPTER TWO COSMETICS IN ANTIQUITY:
THE MIDDLE EAST

Herodotus. Trans. A. D. Godley (1920)

Levey, Martin. *Chemistry and Chemical Technology in Ancient Mesopotamia* (Elsevier Publishing Company, USA 1959)

Lindsay, Jack. *Cleopatra* (1970)

Lucas, A. *Ancient Egyptian Materials and Industries* (1962)

Noblecourt, Christiane Desroches. *Tutankhamun* (1972)

Pound, Ezra and Stock, Noel. *Love Poems of Ancient Egypt* (1962)

Saggs, H. W. F. *Everyday Life in Babylonia and Assyria* (1965)

CHAPTER THREE COSMETICS IN ANTIQUITY:
GREECE AND ROME

Carcopino, Jerome. *Daily Life in Ancient Rome* (1956)

Cowell, F. R. *Everyday Life in Ancient Rome* (1966)

Homer. *The Iliad.* trans into prose by C. W. Bateman and R. Mongan (1860)

Ovid. *Ars Amatoria* trans J. L. May (1959)

Pliny. *Epistles* trans William Melmoth (1925)

Theophrastus. *Enquiry into Plants* trans Sir Arthur Hort (1926)

Willetts, R. F. *Everyday Life in Ancient Crete* (1969)

CHAPTER FOUR EARLY BRITAIN AND THE MIDDLE AGES

Brooke, Iris. *English Costume of the Early Middle Ages* (1936)

—— *English Costume of the Late Middle Ages* (1936)

Chaucer. *The Canterbury Tales*

—— *The Romaunt of the Rose*

Chronicles of the Crusades. Recorded by Richard of Devizes; Geoffrey de Vinsauf and Lord John de Joinville; Henry G. Bohn (1848)

Cockayne, Rev Oswald. *Leechdoms, Wortcunning and Starcraft* (1866)

Coulton, G. G. *The Medieval Scene* (Cambridge University Press 1930)

—— *Life in the Middle Ages* (Cambridge University Press 1928)

Davie, Adam *King Alisaunder* (A thirteenth-century Romance)

Harrison, Michael. *The History of the Hat* (1960)

The Book of the Knight of La Tour Landry trans from the original French in the reign of Henry VI and edited from the unique manuscript in the British Museum by Thomas Wright (Early English Text Society 1868)

Manners and Household Expenses of England in the thirteenth and fifteenth centuries including Manorial Rolls of Eleanor, Countess of Leicester; Expenses of Sir John Howard (1462-9) Roxburghe Club Collection, British Museum

Myers, A. R. *England in the Late Middle Ages* (1952)

Norton, Thomas. *The Ordinall of Alchemy* (fifteenth century)

Paston. *Letters*

Rosenberg, Melrich V. *Eleanor of Aquitaine* (1937)

Russell, John. *The Boke of Nurture* (Roxburghe Club Collection, British Museum. 1460)

Scrope, Stephen. *The Boke of Knyghthode* (Roxburghe Club Collection, British Museum, 1368 trans from the French by Stephen Scrope in the fifteenth century)

Trevelyan, G. M. *Illustrated English Social History* (1944)

William of Malmesbury. *The History of the Kings of England and of His Own Times*, trans Rev John Sharpe (1854)

CHAPTER FIVE THE LATE FIFTEENTH AND SIXTEENTH CENTURIES

Castiglione, Count Baldassare. *The Book of the Courtier*, trans Sir Thomas Hoby (1561)

Cunnington, Cecil Willett. *Handbook of English Costume in the Sixteenth Century* (1962)

Dee, Dr John. *Diary* (sixteenth century)

Della Casa. *Galateo* trans R. S. Pine-Coffin (1958)

Jenkins, Elizabeth. *Elizabeth the Great* (1958)

Ben Jonson. Plays

Neale, Sir John Ernest. *Queen Elizabeth 1st* (1967)

Pater, Walter. *The Renaissance* (1961)

Platt, Sir Hugh. *Delightes For Ladies* (1602)

Shakespeare. Plays and Sonnets

Sidney, Sir Philip. Poems

Vaughn, William. *Naturall and Artificial Directions for Health* (1600)

Wilson, Violet A. *Queen Elizabeth's Maids of Honour and Ladies of the Privy Chamber* (1922)

—— *Society Women in Shakespeare's Time* (1924)

Wright, Thomas. *Queen Elizabeth and her Times*: A series of contemporary Letters (1938)

CHAPTER SIX THE SEVENTEENTH CENTURY

Ashley, Maurice. *Life in Stuart England* (1964)

Crawford, G. M. *Louise de Keroualle, Duchess of Portsmouth* (1887)

Cunnington, Cecil Willett. *Handbook of English Costume in the Seventeenth Century* (1963)

Davidson, Lillias Cambell. *Catherine of Braganza* (1908)

Dowell, Stephen. *A History of Taxation and Taxes in England* (1884)

Etherege, Sir George. *The Man of Mode* (1684)

Evelyn, John. *Diary* (1818)

Norman, Charles. *Rake Rochester* (1955)

Pepys, Samuel. *Diary* (Dent ed 1924)

Savile, Sir George, Marquis of Halifax. *The Lady's New Year Gift or Advice to a Daughter* (1696)

Taylor, Jeremy. *Several Letters Between Two Ladies* (1701)

The Lady's Dressing Room Unlock'd and The Fop's Dictionary (1700)

Thomson, Gladys Scott. *Life in a Noble Household* (1937)

Verney, Frances Parthenope. *Memoirs of the Verney Family* (1892)

CHAPTER SEVEN THE EIGHTEENTH CENTURY

Bleackley, H. W. *The Story of a Beautiful Duchess* (1907)
—— *The Beautiful Duchess* (1927)
Cunnington, Cecil Willett. *Handbook of English Costume in the Eighteenth Century* (1964)
Halsband, Robert. *The Life of Lady Mary Wortley Montagu* (Clarendon Press, Oxford, 1956)
—— *The Complete Letters of Lady Mary Wortley Montagu* (Oxford University Press, 1965)
Laver, James. *English Costume of the Eighteenth Century* (1931)
Pope, Alexander. Poems
Steele, Sir Richard. *The Tatler* (Everyman Library, 1968)
Thomas, E. Wynne. *The House of Yardley* (1953)
Walpole, Horace. *Selected Letters* (1967)

CHAPTER EIGHT THE NINETEENTH CENTURY

Angeloglou, Maggie. *A History of Make-Up* (1970)
Anon. *The Art of Beauty* (1825)
Anon. *The Art of Beauty: A Book for Women and Girls* (1899)
Beerbohm, Max. *In Defence of Cosmetics* (1922)
Cooley, A. J. *The Toilet and Cosmetic Arts* (1866)
Dickens, Charles. Novels
Dudley, Ernest. *The Gilded Lily* (1958)
Elliott, Blanche B. *A History of English Advertising* (1962)
Franzero, Carlo Maria. *The Life and Times of Beau Brummell* (1958)

Piesse, G. W. Septimus. *The Art of Perfumery* (1855)

'Peter Pindar'. Complete Works (1816)

Priestley, J. B. *The Prince of Pleasure* (1969)

Rachel, Madame. *Beautiful For Ever* (1863); 'The Extraordinary
   Life and Times of Madame Rachel' (*Times*, September 1868)

Richardson, Joanne. *Sarah Bernhardt* (1959)

Terry, Ellen. *The Story of My Life* (1908)

Tisdall, E. E. P. *Queen Victoria's Private Life* (1961)

Toilet Table Talk (1856)

Watson, Vera. *A Queen at Home* (1952)

Wilde, Oscar. Plays

CHAPTER NINE THE TWENTIETH CENTURY (1899-1945)

Beaton, Cecil. *The Book of Beauty* (1930)

—— *The Glass of Fashion* (1954)

Coward, Noël. *Private Lives* (1930)

Garland, Madge. *The Indecisive Decade* (1968)

Joyce, Max Wykes. *Cosmetics and Adornment* (1961)

Strauss, Rita. *The Beauty Book* (1924)

Vogue Book of Beauty (1933)

CHAPTER TEN THE TWENTIETH CENTURY (1945-1970s)

Harper's Bazaar Folio of Fashion and Beauty (1949)

Vogue Beauty Book (1948)

Vogue's New Beauty Book (1958-9)

PERIODICALS

Harper's Bazaar (twentieth century)

The Gentleman's Magazine (eighteenth century)

The Ladies' Magazine (eighteenth century)

The Ladies' Journal (nineteenth century)

The Ladies' Pocket Journal (nineteenth century)

BIBLIOGRAPHY

The Tatler (eighteenth century)
Vogue (twentieth century)

EXHIBITIONS

'Chaucer's London' (London Museum, 1972)
'The Masque of Beauty' (National Portrait Gallery, 1972)
'Vanity Through the Ages' (Brighton Museum and Art Gallery,
    1972)

Acknowledgements

I should like to express my sincere gratitude to all those who have helped me in writing this book. Help has been freely forthcoming from a number of sources, but I am particularly indebted to the following museums, organisations and individuals for their kind co-operation:

The Brighton Museum and Art Galley: particularly Mrs Betty O'Looney, exhibitions organiser for the museum's exhibition of 'Vanity through the Ages', for supplying me with so much valuable information on the individual exhibits. The British Museum: especially the staff of the print room for helping me with my picture research. The Victoria and Albert Museum. The British Theatre Museum. The National Gallery. The National Portrait Galley: my thanks are due to the publications department for their interest and help in suggesting suitable paintings to illustrate this book. The Bodleian Library. Condé Nast Publications Ltd. Gerald Duckworth Ltd: I am grateful for their co-operation and should also like to thank two of their authors, Professor James C. Faris and Dr Andrew Strathern for allowing me to reproduce photographs from their books, *Nuba Personal Art* and *Self-Decoration in Mount Hagen*. Yardley and Co Ltd: the staff of their factory at Basildon, Essex, were kind enough to escort me round the factory and patiently answered all my questions. Yardley's London office supplied me with much valuable historical information about the company and the history of cosmetic compounds. Elizabeth Arden Ltd: they too helped in providing me with information on the company and allowed me to reproduce one of their early advertisements in this book. Barbara Attenborough

189

ACKNOWLEDGEMENTS

Associates. Boots and Co Ltd. Cyclax Ltd. Gala of London
Ltd. John R. Freeman and Co Ltd: their team of museum
photographers supplied me with many excellent photographs
of historical material from the British Museum, The Victoria
and Albert Museum and the British Theatre Museum. Miss
Diana Hibling: my sincere thanks to her for patiently typing
the text of the book from my manuscript. I should also like
to thank my brother, Ronnie, for being kind enough to compile
the index, and my husband, Anthony, for all his helpful advice
and sustained interest in this project.

F.G.

Index

191